ZEN CANCER WISDOM

ZEN CANCER WISDOM

. . .

Tips for Making
Each Day Better

Daju Suzanne Friedman

WISDOM PUBLICATIONS • BOSTON

Wisdom Publications
199 Elm Street
Somerville MA 02144 USA
www.wisdompubs.org

Library of Congress Cataloging-in-Publication Data
Friedman, Daju Suzanne.
  Zen cancer wisdom : tips for making each day better / Daju Suzanne Friedman.
    pages cm
  ISBN 1-61429-123-3 (pbk. : alk. paper)
  1. Cancer—Alternative treatment. 2. Cancer—Patients—Life skills guides. 3. Cancer—Religious aspects—Zen Buddhism. 4. Spiritual life—Zen Buddhism. I. Title.
  RC271.A62F75 2014
  616.99'4—dc23
                              2014005498
ISBN 9781614291237   ebook ISBN 9781614291466

18 17 16 15 14
5 4 3 2 1

Cover design by Phil Pascuzzo. Illustrations by Andy Francis.
Interior design by Gopa&Ted2, Inc. Set in Whitman 11.25/16.

Wisdom Publications' books are printed on acid-free paper and meet the guidelines for permanence and durability of the Production Guidelines for Book Longevity of the Council on Library Resources.

This book was produced with environmental mindfulness. We have elected to print this title on 30% PCW recycled paper. As a result, we have saved the following resources: 19 trees, 9 million BTUs of energy, 1,658 lbs. of greenhouse gases, 8,991 gallons of water, and 602 lbs. of solid waste. For more information, please visit our website, www.wisdompubs.org.

Printed in the United States of America.

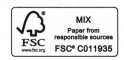

For more information, please visit www.fscus.org.

"When one has understanding,
one should laugh; one should not weep."
—HSUEH TOU

· · ·

"If you have lost your sense of humor
you have lost your way."
—JUNPO KELLY ROSHI

• • •

To my family, for their incredible love, support, optimism, and laughter.

To my Zen master and dear friend, Junpo Denis Kelly Roshi. The heart energy of the master and that of the pupil fit like a box and its lid.

To my healing team: Garrett Smith, Michael Broffman, Linda Asbury, Peggy Arent, Brain Weissbuch, Anna Dorian, Brian LaForgia, Jacob Chinn, Christy Mahoney, Vadim Derevyanko, Mark Renneker, Deb Follingstad, and Robert Nagourney.

To Andy Francis, my editor at Wisdom Publications. You are truly a wish-fulfilling jewel.

And most especially, to Suzannah Margaret Stason, my every-flower. Your love, kindness, compassion, and presence are the strongest medicines I've ever encountered. I am grateful for every moment with you.

• • •

Contents

V. Self-Healing Qigong Exercises

Foreword

CANCER. What a wake-up call! You now have a direct realization of the truth of impermanence. What are you going to do? Don't waste another moment! Having cancer has been like an enormously interesting Technicolor 3-D movie. It didn't matter whether I liked it or not; it happened. Still, when I consider it from a deeper perspective, I wouldn't have missed it or any of the other so-called "awful" circumstances in my life.

Zen is the Japanese word for insight, awareness, and meditative mind. Zen is practiced to resolve the great confusion about life and death. If we see life and death as the same continuous process, we can fully experience life as a great gift. The ego wants comfort and permanence and freedom from pain. But when we can't have those, what do we do? How do we open ourselves to what is in front of us? We don't get to choose our experiences, but we can choose how we respond to them. Zen practice reveals that intelligence is brighter than our passions, our emotions. We can learn to stay fiercely and intelligently present or we can spin out into confusion.

I was shocked when I was diagnosed with cancer. I had

been a longtime Zen practitioner and Ashtangi yogi, eating right and living right, and then there was a lump in my neck: Stage IV oropharangeal (a.k.a. throat) cancer. I actually thought the way I lived would protect me from old age and death! Then cancer came calling . . . Wake up!

Meditation practice, along with allowing me to be present with what is—with whatever is arising—allowed me to observe the cancer as "interesting" (not in a happy way, mind you). I consulted with doctors far and wide to find what might work to cure it. I did complementary medicine as well as intensive radiation and heavy chemotherapy. When my doc first saw me, he said that I looked like I "could take a punch" and decided he would go after it with the big guns. It worked.

I joke now that, like Woody Allen, I don't fear death; I fear life! I'm fundamental in my Buddhist view, but an agnostic in general. I don't concern myself with what's next. The ego is a temporary construct, and when you have cancer you finally "get" impermanence. You get a taste of the truth of what Zen calls "nonexistence"—the truth that your socially constructed ego is not who you really are. "How extraordinarily interesting! How difficult!" This is the Zen view.

The side effects of treatment can get quite noisy. The gift that Zen practice gives is the ability to stay with what is. It isn't to become passive or nihilistic. We remain critically intelligent, paying full attention to what is happening, and trying to do what is necessary. What are our choices? Do we choose to live from a broader Zen perspective that transcends mental chatter, pain, and suffering? If we can do that, then in the face of any type of insult intelligence and discernment will prevail over emotionality and self-referencing. The gift of Zen that this book brings is the ability to stay conscious and present throughout the course of cancer.

I put my cancer where it belongs, behind me. I returned fully to life. I still eat well and practice Zen and yoga. The question for us all is, "What do we do with the rest of our lives?" For me, the answer was to go back to work. People are suffering. What is it for you?

I spread the Zen view and insight that our angst is our liberation. The practice is to stay conscious and awake in the face of whatever is, because we are, in essence, conscious awareness. We are only secondarily an ego— evaluative, interpretive, and constantly self-referencing. When we stand in the light as the light, witnessing life from this deep perspective, we notice how extraordinarily interesting everything is, and how karmically interrelated and interconnected everything is. How could it be otherwise? Life is going to unfold as it will.

So now what?

If you are new to Zen or meditation, I recommend that you begin with some of the breathing exercises in this book. They will help prepare you for concentration meditation, such as counting while you sit (also included in this book). You will learn how to breathe into the space deeper and broader than your mind or thoughts. From this depth, you can experience fear and release it. This book will help you to feel better on many levels—physical, emotional, and spiritual. Each level matters, and each is adequately addressed.

I have practiced many of the tips in this book, and they work. But remember: each tip is like a finger pointing at the moon. It can show you the way but you can get there only through your own efforts, through your own unique personal practice. Do not waste another moment!

Junpo Kando Denis Kelly Roshi
Abbot, Hollow Bones Zen Order
Appleton, Wisconsin

Introduction

I WROTE THIS BOOK to wake you up, shake you up, and hopefully, at times, even to crack you up as you walk the path of cancer. It was written as much for me as it was for you. The majority of this book was written during my first and second cycles of chemotherapy for a recurrence of Stage IV lung cancer.

My story is just like yours—unique and not unique. I'm a Zen priest, Chinese medicine doctor, and qigong master. When I was forty-one years old I was diagnosed with Stage IV lung cancer despite having lived the life of a meticulous health nut for over twenty years. The cancer went into remission after six months of non-chemo pharmaceuticals and an extensive complementary medicine regimen. It came back almost a year later, when I was forty-three. After trying everything else, I began chemotherapy and fortified my complementary medicine regimen to address the effects—ahem, I mean "side effects"—of the chemo.

I went from a Chinese medicine doctor whose practice focused on cancer patients to a cancer patient myself. The world didn't make sense anymore. I was living the ultimate Zen koan or riddle: How could my anticancer lifestyle have led to Stage IV lung cancer? How could true love, broccoli, and qigong lead to illness? Zen is about fiercely facing what is in front of you, not about looking longingly behind you.

Layman Wang once asked his attendant, "What would you do if a dragon suddenly arrived here?" His attendant answered, "I wouldn't pay attention to anything else." This is how it feels when you've been diagnosed with cancer. Your attention and focus shift dramatically toward just this one thing. While single-minded focus can be beneficial, it is also important to remember that you are more than your diagnosis and that there is more to life than being a patient.

I decided early on that I wouldn't let cancer take away my sense of humor or my *joie d'vivre*. I experimented and discovered firsthand exactly what helped or hindered my mood, energy, body, and/or spirit. I learned how to ease unnecessary suffering during my cancer journey and began sharing this information with friends, family, patients, and strangers.

Why include spiritual Zen with practical complementary cancer approaches? Because Buddhism is unique in its head-on approach to suffering, and Zen is all about the practical art of living, rather than some abstract philosophy to ponder and master. What is Zen? Zen is the act of giving yourself over to this moment, to being fully present in your life. This book is about the Zen of healing.

Each entry presents a special thought, action, or opportunity to make this and each day better. There is no correct order, so you can open to any page for some food for thought, sage advice, or a quick and dirty healing tip.

Master Jiashan once said that swarming fish don't notice the pearl in the dragon's mouth. They're too distracted by the dragon to see the pearl. This too applies when you or a loved one has cancer. It is easy for the dragons of cancer to overshadow and even obscure the pearls on this journey.

They say the best a Zen teacher can do is point her finger toward the moon; to point you in the right direction. With that in mind, it is my sincere hope that this book points you toward the pearls on this path. No matter how dark it gets, the moon is always there. Sometimes we could use a gentle reminder or practice to get us back on track. With any luck, there should be something in here that will do that for you.

The purpose of all the tips in this book is to help you feel better now, and if not now, then at least quickly or soon. There is one catch: you must actually try them! Reading this book without practicing its contents is like reading the label on a medicine bottle but not taking the medicine. You know what's inside, but how can it help you from inside the bottle? Take the medicine and see for yourself!

What are you waiting for? Waiting is so not Zen. It's time to grab the tiger by the whiskers!

A Note Regarding the Names of Zen Masters

In Japan and America, Zen masters are usually known by their Japanese names, even when the master is Chinese. For example, Linji, a Chinese Zen master, is better known by his Japanese name, Rinzai. Master Zhaozhou is better known as Joshu. This text uses the true Chinese names of every Zen master mentioned, and presents each name in pinyin romanization.

Pronunciation Guide for Pinyin

Vowels:

ao is pronounced *ow* as in "cow."
ou is pronounced *oe* as in "row."
a is pronounced *ah* as in "car."
o is pronounced *oo* as in "look."
ui is pronounced *uay* as in "way."
e is pronounced *uh* as in "thumb."
i after compound consonants is *r*, therefore *shi* and *zhi* are pronounced *shr* and *zhr*.
i after single consonants is pronounced *ee* as in "bee."

Consonants:

x is pronounced *sh* as in "share."

q is pronounced *ch* as in "cherry."

zh is pronounced *j* as in "joke." (For easier reading, this text sometimes substitutes a *j* for *zh* in names).

c is pronounced *ts* as in "rats."

I.
Practical Navigation Wisdom

1.

Learning Is Not the Path

HOW MUCH IS ENOUGH INFORMATION?

Master Nanquan taught that the life path is to be
"experienced," not merely spent accumulating knowledge.

YOU ONLY HAVE so much time in a day. How can you
best spend your time, your most precious resource? This
question is applicable, at any time, regardless of circumstances. In Zen, experience and insight are valued more
highly than the information we have stored between our
ears. Master Nanquan valued full engagement in life over
spending his days studying about it. For example, we
could spend all of our free time reading book after book
about meditation and its benefits, or we could sit down
and actually meditate. Which is best for experiencing the
truth of who we are?

The same holds true when it comes to approaching
your cancer diagnosis or the cancer diagnosis of a loved
one. The learning curve is truly ridiculous; you are given
no time to make what can likely be the most important
decisions of your life (Here's where I urge you to keep

9

in mind that it gets much easier once this phase is taken care of). So how do you begin? Begin right where you are. Breathe. And get whatever help you need to make the most informed decision you can, given the circumstances.

You will undoubtedly learn much on this journey. Some of us choose to learn more about cancer in general or about our particular type of cancer. Others may not do any research at all. It isn't necessary to become a specialist. There are plenty of specialists out there willing to talk with you. Find them and use them when you need them!

Yes, learning is important. But understanding is even more important when it comes to making decisions about cancer care. We might take the question "When is enough information enough?" as our koan (a challenging riddle used in Zen contemplation). How would we answer this? Are we chasing information simply to make ourselves more comfortable, or do we already have enough to make an informed decision? Check in with yourself.

If you have a background in research, like me, you may go nuts trying to learn about every available option in order to make the most informed decisions. But rest assured that there will always be further information out there. Find out what the best resources are for your questions and use them when you need to. This will relieve some unnecessary pressure and tension that we may hold inside. For example, during my own search for answers, I found a local doctor who keeps up with cutting-edge cancer approaches. He does phone consultations, and I contact him for a second opinion whenever I need to make a change in my treatment protocol. I also have a local Chinese medicine doctor and cancer researcher who knows more about cancer research than anyone else I've ever encountered. These two docs save me hours I would have spent reading through studies and the latest publications. There are many people out there who offer these services. Find the ones with whom you resonate and use them for all they're worth!

We can research like crazy. It is up to us to find the balance between the energy expended on research and its potential benefits for our healing path. Once you get the important questions answered, check in with yourself to see if what you have is enough. Years ago I had a patient who spent month after month gathering various opinions from all over the country, and he ended up with so many conflicting choices that he couldn't make a choice. The information weighed him down to the point where it was no longer useful. How many opinions will you need before you feel ready to embark on a treatment plan? Who are the best doctors for your particular issues? Where is the best place for this type of treatment? And of course my favorite: What lifestyle approaches can help keep you grounded and address potential treatment side effects? (Hint: many are in this book!)

Knowledge is power, but healing is the path.

2.

A Head Like a Coconut

REMEMBERING THE IMPORTANT STUFF

There was once a Chinese governor famous for
having read thousands of scriptures. The governor
found himself to be most impressive. Zen Master
Guizhong did not. He teasingly asked how all those
scriptures could fit into the governor's head, which
was only about the size of a coconut.

IN MY PAST LIFE as a lawyer I learned just how faulty
people's memories can be. We are all witnesses to our own
lives; witnesses with a finite amount of reliable memory
available to us; witnesses with coconut heads. Studies
show that we tend to think we will remember more, and
more accurately, than we really do. But our heads are only
so big, after all!

It would take someone with a rare gift to be able to
remember all of the fancy medical terms and the names
of medicines you will be introduced to on this journey.
Add "chemo brain" into the mix and watch as the things

you were sure you'd remember disappear without a trace into the brain fog.

Be gentle with yourself when this happens. This experience is one big exercise in letting go of the illusion of control. Since you are a mere mortal, it is perfectly natural to mess up, to forget, and to ask for help and support when you need it. Other mere mortals are here for you and they want to help. In fact, they are patiently waiting for you to ask, I guarantee it.

Keeping this in mind, if at all possible, bring a friend or a family member to all of your doctor appointments. That person will be in charge of writing down what's important while you pay attention to what's happening during the conversation. It is so much easier to pay attention when thoughts like "I'd better remember this!" aren't echoing over and over through our coconut-like heads.

If you can't find yourself a second pair of eyes and ears, then you might purchase a cheap digital recorder, use the voice memo function on your cell phone, or take notes at the appointment. Find what feels easiest for you. Some people relax better when they have more to do. If this sounds like you, perhaps writing the information down yourself would be best.

Writing things down or recording them means we will have the correct information whenever we need it. Keep your information in a safe, accessible place, just in case.

You now have the perfect opportunity to practice the

art of asking for help. Don't be hard-headed—you only have so much memory in your head's hard drive. When it comes to visits to doctors, phone calls from doctors, or whenever you know you'll need to retain important information, remember that two heads are better than one!

3.

Not-Knowing Mind

STAYING OPEN TO OPTIONS

"Not-knowing mind," also called beginner's mind,
includes all possibilities. The beginner, not yet aware
of limitations, has an open and infinite view.

WHEN WE ARE OPEN to infinite possibility, our options greatly increase. The more we explore, the more there is in our awareness, the more there is from which to pick and choose. When I was a student in Chinese medicine school, a seasoned teacher once said that he envied beginning practitioners, because we beginners were still willing to be more daring and to take chances with our treatment protocols.

Beginners don't play it safe; they are not yet set in their ways or shut down to untraveled pathways. Beginners don't yet have a comfort zone beyond which they are afraid to venture. Beginners practice the art of "not-knowing mind," which means that because they know that they don't know, they are willing to try just about anything. In spite of the fear that comes with not having all the answers, we gain a certain freedom when we embrace not knowing.

Cancer can certainly challenge our well-worn beliefs, but this challenge also provides us the opportunity to open ourselves more fully to life. We engage more fully with what's around us when we release stale, old, limiting beliefs. Well-worn patterns of thought take us down familiar, oft-travelled roads. Cancer pushes us to do a little off-road exploration. You game?

More options. That sounds pretty darn good to this cancer patient. I can't tell you how many things I've done that I never thought I'd do before cancer came along. If there's one thing I have truly learned from cancer, it is that you never know what might happen, and you never know how you are going to respond to what happens until it happens. Although I didn't ask to be shocked into not-knowing mind, I have come to relish the freedom and openness that it brings. I find that the not-knowing mind applies just as much to my daily life as it did to my approach to cancer care.

Zen teachers often warn us not to believe our thoughts and to get out of our own way. Cancer, like an ornery Zen master, gives us a strong incentive to get out of our own way. It forces us to leave behind resentment of what cannot be and to open ourselves to every possibility. We may never have considered foreign medical traditions before, but millions and millions of people have been using systems like Indian Ayurveda or traditional Chinese medicine to treat cancer and other diseases for thousands and thousands of years. We may never have thought about how each piece of food we put into our bodies contributes to our overall health. There may in fact be something in complementary medical traditions that works right for you. There may in fact be foods that can help offset nutritional deficiencies caused by your treatments. Be open to the possibilities, and find professionals with expertise in these areas to be best informed about them.

- Drop your agenda, opinions, and prejudice when evaluating possibilities.
- Let go of the thought "I know, I know," and approach things with the fresh and open mind of a beginner.
- When you feel your mind contracting and closing itself off to a particular possibility, recognize that you can choose to set aside preconceptions and remain open to it.
- Make a habit of this recognition, and understand that "I know, I know" is often a habitual response grounded in fear of the unknown rather than in real knowledge.
- When the skeptical thought "I don't know" arises, allow that not-knowing to become curiosity.
- Make a habit of letting curiosity rise to meet the possibilities that you feel suspicious or dismissive of, but don't actually know much about.

You can practice this not-knowing mind with regard to the little things in life, as well as the big! Anything is possible . . . unless you disagree!

4.

Flawless Jade

LOOKING GOOD, REGARDLESS

The I-Ching, an ancient Chinese divination manual,
says that sometimes we should decorate or beautify
our outer appearance as a way of reflecting our
inner beauty and worth.

LET'S BE HONEST: how you look can influence, for better or for worse, how you feel about yourself. If your feelings of self-worth have taken a hit (or two, or three), this one's for you.

Master Panshan wisely pointed out that when jade is concealed within stone, "the stone has no knowledge of the jade's flawless nature." Sometimes it is impossible to see the truth of one's inner nature—of what lies beneath the surface. Though we may be particularly skilled at judging and comparing ourselves to others, we sometimes lose sight of our intrinsic value—the truth of who we are, concealed deep within us. We see only rough stone on the outside, but not the flawless jade hidden on the inside. It is especially true that during cancer we are apt to lose sight of or forget our beautiful, untouchable, flawless inner nature.

It is time to remember and get in touch with your inner beauty. If you look in the mirror these days and wonder who the heck is staring back at you, just remember that the flawless jade of who you are inside cannot be touched or marred by the way you appear on the outside. I remind myself of this regularly.

When I was undergoing chemo, I decided that every time I went I would wear my fancy jade and pearl mala (rosary) necklace that has a jade pendant carved into the Chinese character for longevity. Of course I liked the way it looked, but I also felt that it helped protect me some-how, like a good luck charm. It also added a touch of fancy to my otherwise bland appearance.

- Consider what you might do with how you look to make yourself feel more powerful, or at least more comfortable with how you appear to others. Any-thing can serve as an amulet, or good luck charm— get creative! Try a lucky shirt, a fabulous hat, or a piece of jewelry that has special meaning. Anna, one of my dearest friends, got a big henna tattoo on her bald head. She looked absolutely beautiful. A favor-ite watch, a favorite pair of shoes, or a scent you are fond of can make a big difference in your day.
- When was the last time you got dressed up and went out for a special occasion? You may feel hesitant to

go out and show your face while undergoing treatment. I certainly did. My face took on a dark purple color and was covered in hundreds of tiny whiteheads! Still, I found that the more I went out, the more I remembered who I am inside and came to be okay with how I looked. Call a friend and treat yourself to a special outing.

It is all too easy to let our appearances influence how we feel about ourselves. The truth is that nothing can mar or take away our innate worth, our inner beauty, our flawless nature. We are still who we are regardless of appearances.

Sometimes all it takes is one small step to make a huge difference in how we appear to ourselves and, as a consequence, how we appear to others. Beginning today, choose something to carry or wear that can be an outward display of your courage, your inner beauty, your valor, and your strength! Let the flawless jade of your inner nature shine through.

5.
To Know the Road Ahead, Ask Someone Returning

GETTING ANSWERS TO KEY QUESTIONS

Zhaozhou, when still a Zen master in training,
   asked Master Nanquan, "What is the Way?"
"Everyday mind is the Way," Master Nanquan answered.

MASTER NANQUAN had a knack for using few words to cut right to the very marrow of things. The most straightforward, uncomplicated way is often the way to go. You need nothing more than your everyday mind, nothing more than common sense, when walking your path. Take the advice offered in the Zen phrase "To know the road ahead, ask someone returning." Put the common sense of Master Nanquan's insightful and practical words of wisdom to work by talking to others who have been where you're heading.

You are probably not the first person to have your particular type of cancer. Doing even a quick Internet search will yield an overwhelming amount of information about your cancer, some accurate, some not so much. While the Internet is a great resource, real, live people are often an even greater resource. And they're everywhere! People are reliable and can save you the task of sifting through ridiculous amounts of useless information. Why reinvent the wheel?

- It is easy to network and find someone to talk with who knows firsthand what you are going through. You can call support groups or ask your oncologist to find other patients willing to talk with you on the phone. Other patients are often the best and easiest-to-find resource. Sometimes a few words from a person who's been through what we're going through can put our minds at ease. Find that person.
- If you can't connect with other folks, talk with your oncologist about what he has seen with other people in your situation. Or call or sit down with another oncologist who specializes in your type of cancer and ask for advice based on what she has seen with her own patients.
- Immediately after receiving a diagnosis, during the information-gathering period, and when it is time to change your treatment plan are all good times to hear from others who've been through the process. Sitting down to talk with others is an efficient use of time at such critical junctures.

In my own case, I chose to ask a handful of medical professionals for recommendations based on their experiences. I didn't purposefully seek out other lung cancer patients, but I did, and still do, talk to all kinds of cancer patients almost every day.

The road we have found ourselves on has many beautiful spirits. Find a few willing to share, and watch as your fears are left behind on the trail.

6.

The Expert Archer Does Not Try to Hit the Target

LEARN SOMETHING NEW

An expert archer hits the bull's-eye with what seems like minimal effort. But the ability to make effort look effortless, called wu wei *in Chinese, comes from long hours practice.*

WHEN WE LOSE ourselves in the enjoyment of cultivating a skill or knowledge about a particular subject, we embody "effortless effort." The expert archer no longer "tries" to do anything. The archer, the arrow, and the target are all one. From this viewpoint, how could an archer miss?

A cancer diagnosis does not have to mean withdrawal from living a fully engaged life. Quite the contrary! Cancer—especially if it means being absent from work as you undergo treatment—may even give you the time to pursue interests you ordinarily wouldn't be able to. Spending time doing something you find meaningful will not only make you feel better mentally, it can actually benefit you physically. When we engage in enjoyable self-cultivation, our bodies naturally release feel-good chemicals. Studies show that the effects that positive attitudes and positive action can have on our biochemistry may aid the healing process. So why not include learning and mastering something new in our process of healing? There is absolutely nothing to lose and so much to be gained from engaging in something that brings with it a positive sense of satisfaction.

The art I took up to cultivate "effortless effort" is the art of *shakuhachi*, the Japanese Zen bamboo flute. Playing the shakuhachi soothes my soul, challenges my mind, and strengthens my lungs. I may never become a master, but that's not the point. The shakuhachi offers me the opportunity to lose myself in cultivation of the art, where there is no me, no flute, no tune.

- Perhaps there is a skill you've always wanted to master, like art, photography, or gardening, for example. Or maybe there is a subject you've had an interest in but have never had the time to study, like history, or foreign languages and cultures. Take the time to get in touch with yourself, to recall your neglected interests.
- Do a quick search for any local clubs, classes, or meet-ups related to your interest. Many online book clubs, teaching videos, and classes are either free or very cheaply priced. Connecting with a group of like-minded enthusiasts is a great way to stay connected and get away from letting your cancer define you.

- For those less inclined to pursue a skill or activity socially, there are many skills that can be honed in the comfort of home. Knitting is very big right now. Cooking is a skill that most of us only ever think of as a necessity. Perhaps you have a friend with whom you might regularly meet to prepare and share new, and hopefully healthy, recipes.
- Find an area of your life in which to cultivate your own effortless effort . . . then do it.

The study or practice of something you love can help you to heal. It can help you to heal physically, emotionally, or spiritually. Each of these aspects of healing are important, and often when you address one the others will also be affected, as they are all interconnected.

When absorbed in practice or study, we truly embrace the moment. We are no longer cancer patients; we become effortless effort. Where there was an arrow and a target, suddenly there is only a bull's-eye.

7.

Empty Your Cup!

BEING FLEXIBLE

A know-it-all visited Zen Master Nan-in to see if there was
anything left worth learning. When Nan-in poured tea for
the man, he kept pouring until the cup overflowed.
"It's too full, no more will go in!" the man shouted.
Nan-in coolly replied, "You are like this cup: full of opinions.
How can I teach you Zen unless you empty your cup?"

HUMILITY, OPENNESS, and sometimes even ignorance can be assets when you are sorting through treatment options. Before cancer I wouldn't even take an aspirin because it "wasn't natural." Since cancer I have taken the strongest lab-made pharmaceuticals out there. Cancer grabbed my cup and turned it upside down. I am now considerably more open-minded when reviewing my options.

The sages were right: it is most beneficial to be like bamboo—strong yet flexible, bending in response to the winds around us.

What feels right initially may not pan out, and what seems crazy now may seem not so crazy later. Your tastes will naturally change and evolve as you grow. Are you willing to pour out what is no longer useful?

Keep your cup empty throughout this journey and you'll maximize the chances of getting it filled in just the right way—over and over again.

8.

Beware the Three-Inch Scholar

FIND THE EXPERTS

*"Beware the three-inch scholar." This Zen expression
is a warning about people who read or hear something
and then talk about it as if they were experts. Their mastery
of the subject was as long and arduous as the three inches
it took the information to get from their eyes or ears,
when they read or heard about it, to their mouths.*

SURELY I WON'T BE the only one to have gotten email
after email about the newest and best cancer cures from
well-meaning folks after they learned of my diagnosis.
If random acquaintances were sending these kinds of
emails to me—a doctor of Chinese medicine with ten
years of experience treating cancer patients—I can only
imagine what others have had to sift through after their
own diagnoses.

It is important to appreciate the love and care of our
friends and families, even when that love and care is
expressed as a recommendation to purchase a "cancer
zapping machine," or in the form of information about

the latest Kenyan treatment innovations involving jungle animals. There are many cancer treatments and remedies out there that look good in advertisements, but which lack meaningful studies to back them up. It is perfectly fine to be open to experimentation, but it is important to find a real professional who knows what works and what doesn't before you spend all your time and money on something that is clearly too good to be true.

Medical doctors know about pharmaceuticals. Licensed herbalists know about natural herbs and their properties. Nutritionists know about food, vitamins, and supplements. These people have studied their subjects well and should have the clinical experience to back up their recommendations.

It is always worth it to run a treatment idea or remedy past someone who knows more about it than you or your well-meaning friends. A little bit of knowledge is a dangerous thing. So is an itty-bitty scholar.

Find true scholars for the information you need.

9.

The Supreme Way Is Not Difficult

CHOOSING WHAT FITS

A monk asked Master Shitou, "What is liberation?"
"Who has bound you?" the master asked in reply.

WE ONLY NEED liberation if we are not free. This is great to keep in mind when we forget that we are often the ones putting the most pressure on ourselves. We are ultimately in charge of what we do and of the decisions we make.

Have you tried something that didn't feel quite right, but you felt compelled to keep pushing despite all evidence that you should stop? You likely agree that when something seems too good to be true, it usually is. In Zen, the opposite is also true. If something seems not to be good enough, it usually isn't.

I have tried many experimental treatments and self-healing techniques on my journey. Without fail, the ones that felt the most forced—that took the most effort for the least return—didn't feel worth it in the end. Likewise, those that clicked the best with me often made a positive difference.

There are plenty of things you can do to help your body stay strong and fight. The important thing is to choose those that fit you and who you are. Being a cancer patient involves enough drama in itself. Who needs more? No drama.

There will always be someone who takes more vitamins than you do, who exercises more than you do, who meditates more than you do. Good for them. They are not your business; you are.

In Zen, we say "the supreme way is not difficult." When you find your supreme way—the way that feels the most fitting and natural to you—it is like ice dissolving into cool, flowing water. If what you are doing to help yourself is not working, or if your efforts have been bearing little fruit, it may be time for something new. You are free to choose new options at any time.

What are you bound by?

10.
Without Words, Without Silence

REACHING OUT TO OTHERS

Here is a real Zen koan, or riddle:
How does one show up without words, but also without
silence?
With one's actions.

FEW PEOPLE KNOW what the hell to say when you have cancer, but most want to help in some way. Excessive pride and cancer are like sushi and red wine—they just don't go together. If no one has said this yet, let me be the first:

YOU HAVE CANCER. ASK FOR HELP!

Besides dealing with the cancer itself, you may also have to rely on others to help with simple things like food preparation, shopping, or even getting dressed. Before cancer, I had a hard time receiving even small kindnesses, and I rarely asked for favors. After cancer, I still have a hard time asking and receiving, but I've gotten better at it out of necessity.

We have all given someone a helping hand. It feels good. Why not let our loved ones feel good, or at least useful? Helping empowers our friends and gives them an opportunity to be of service, to contribute to our healing in some small or large way. It is a gift that benefits the giver as much as the receiver. The act of giving becomes a win-win situation. You both feel better.

When we give people an opportunity to help, we give them a chance to express their care and love with actions, rather than with words. The messages in our hearts are best conveyed by actions anyway; words often fail. Your friends and family members want to show their support.

If people offer to help, accept it. Find something meaningful for them to do. It will help them feel better too.

11.

Do Not Fight with Another's Bow and Arrow

FOLLOWING YOUR OWN PATH

Do not fight with another's bow and arrow!
Do not ride another's horse!
Do not discuss another's faults.
Do not interfere with another's work.

THIS POEM from Wumen's commentary to *The Gateless Gate*, a classic book of koans, is not just wise advice; it is a wise way to live. Simply stated, he is exhorting us to find our own way and to leave the ways of others to themselves.

Deciding on a treatment plan is rarely a breeze. Peace of mind comes from understanding what's happening and knowing all of your options so that the treatment plan you choose is the right one for you. What is right for someone else, whether it has worked or not, may not be right for you, and that's just fine.

Ask whatever questions you have when making decisions. Don't be shy when it comes to asking doctors each and every question you have. Your treatment is your bow and arrow or your companion horse. Picture the difference between riding a horse you've come to understand and know, and jumping on a wild stallion you've never seen before. Cancer is already a wild enough ride!

Arm yourself with whatever knowledge you need to feel comfortable with making a decision. Sometimes you may get lucky and there will be one clear way to go. More often, you will be presented with multiple options, each with its own pros and cons. A treatment plan that you are comfortable with, one that will allow you at least some small sense of peace of mind—that's your target.

Some choose an integrative approach, such as the one put forth in this book. Others choose to do only chemotherapy, surgery, and/or radiation. An even smaller group will choose exclusively alternative and complementary medicine as their bow and arrow. There is no "one size fits all" approach to cancer care. You may need to try out a few different approaches before you find the one that suits you. It is worth it to experiment until you find your way.

The treatment of cancer is an art as well as a science. There are doctors who approach their treatments in black and white, and others whose approach involves more nuances and colors. Discover what you feel more comfortable with by asking all of the questions that help put your mind at ease.

Likewise, other patients may have settled on different treatment routes. Good for them. If you have questions, ask them; otherwise, follow Wumen's advice and choose the bow and arrow and horse that suit you best.

You should feel a nice sense of accomplishment once you have decided on a treatment plan. After a plan is in place, so much of your time and head-space are freed up for other things, like living your life! I often find it a great relief to have settled on an option that feels right to me based on my own knowledge.

May your chosen arrow hit the target and your horse run like the wind.

12.

When Two Thieves Meet, They Need No Introduction

SHARING IN COMMUNITY

There's an old saying: "When two thieves meet, they need no introduction; they recognize each other without question."

SIMILAR NATURES recognize each other. We tend to know whom we're drawn to, if not always why. While it isn't hard to recognize our own kind, it may be tricky to find them.

Have you looked into a support group yet? Good support groups are worth seeking out, because the more you feel an affinity with the people in the group, the better you'll feel. It's that simple, really.

A support group, particularly one with the right mix of people, can be invaluable. Support groups are a great resource for tips from people who have already been through what you are going through or about to go through.

If a support group is not your thing, try taking an art

class, or pursuing a hobby, like birding, photography, or woodworking, with a local group of hobbyists. Not ringing your bell? Invite old friends to come over for tea. Make it a regular thing. Or, if you'd prefer, go on a walk with someone special (besides your pooch). Make it a regular thing. Having hobbies and routines—actively choosing positive ways to spend our time—is an asset in life as well as in healing.

Being around people who interest us is an easy way to keep our minds focused, calm, and in the present, where things are usually not as bad as you fear they could be. Where are your people? Where can you share openly in a supportive environment with folks who "get you"? Ask around. Don't let shyness stop you. Lots of people in support groups and activity groups are shy.

13.
The Build Goodness Temple

WELCOMING THE POSITIVE

*"Build Goodness Temple" is really the name
of an old Chinese Zen temple. The name reflects
the goal of its residents.*

THE PURPOSE of this temple has really stuck with me, and I've come to see my daily life as a sort of "build goodness temple." I've chosen to surround myself with people who add goodness and meaning to my days. I choose activities that feel like donations to my personal "build goodness temple," such as tea dates with friends and walks with my two little dogs along the beach.

If someone tries to bring dust into my temple, or something feels like it is taking away from the goodness of my temple, I don't welcome it in. Like a samurai guarding the gate, I see myself trying to prevent or cut entanglements with situations and people that don't serve my greater good.

This is probably one of the easiest tips in this book, as we are often well aware of what brings us a greater feeling of goodness and what just doesn't cut it. If you are not sure of what might help you accumulate more "goodness" in your temple, today is the perfect day to take some time in silence and stillness to tune in to your inner temple guardian.

Have you been tolerating the build-up of dust and debris in your temple? It may be time for a deep cleaning. Sometimes we simply need to clear out the mental clutter to realize that our precious inner space can be better used for something meaningful; something that makes us smile, think, or slow down.

In stillness and silence, slow down and take a look at your state of mind:

How have you been?

How long has it been since you've done a little something to uplift yourself?

Has the craziness of life left you feeling cluttered?

There are many small things that we can do to refresh ourselves and open up a bit of space inside, whether we are at home, at a friend's place, in a hotel, or in a hospital:

- Open the blinds and open the windows to let a little fresh air in.
- A fresh bouquet of flowers for a table or altar adds just the right touch of beauty to help you slow down and smile.

- A visit from an old friend brings cheer and livens up the place.
- Listen to music that lifts your spirits.
- Look at pictures of loved ones or of art that inspires you.
- Make it a regular habit to tidy up the temple of your mind.

When I don't have a ton of energy, I like to lay on the couch and pet my dogs, or even take a nap with a dog on my lap. Slow and easy quality time with loved ones or one's pets is a great rejuvenator.

If you end up staying in the hospital or stuck at home, ask friends or loved ones to help you get whatever you need to create a goodness temple wherever you are. If you are in a hospital and don't have a window, ask if it would be possible to be moved to a room with a window. Here's that theme again: it never hurts to ask! Your friends are eager and waiting to offer a helping hand. Let them help you cultivate a good environment in your home temple, wherever home happens to be at this moment.

It may be more difficult to cut entanglements with people or situations that don't help you feel more goodness in your space. You may have a well-intended friend or family member who brings more worry than support. Limiting your contact with her to email messages may work wonders in this instance. The thing about cancer is that when you tell people you are not in the mood to have visitors, they tend to respect your wishes and rarely push. Use this to your benefit!

Your home is your sanctuary, as is your mind. Welcome in what makes you feel calmer, clearer, and more collected. Be vigilant to bar what clutters, disturbs, and drags you down. You already know the best place to begin: right where you live.

14.

Tame the First Lion

TRYING NEW APPROACHES

*"Tame the first lion well, and the remaining lions
will fall easily into place. If you fail to tame the first lion,
the other lions will learn to remain untamed."*

ZEN DISCIPLINARIANS in China used this metaphor to
explain the importance of getting the first, foundational
step of a process right. Teachers and parents will understand exactly what they were getting at.

Most oncologists would agree that this, too, is their
goal when they decide on a treatment protocol. If they get
it right the first time, the cancer goes away faster and the
patient gets away with less toxicity and overall trauma.
Modern oncology is producing many cutting-edge
approaches that can take live cancer cells or blood on
which to perform ex-vivo tests to see what treatments
will be most effective for that particular cancer. This new
science is just now becoming more well-known outside
of major city centers, so your oncologist may not have
heard of it.

I have reason to thoroughly believe in this approach. When I was first diagnosed, I chose to have surgery to remove a cancerous lymph node, which was sent to a clinical oncologist, who could then test various drugs on my live cancer. Before the surgery, the first oncologist I saw gave me six to seven months to live, but after I started the protocol determined to be most effective according to my lab results, my cancer practically melted away. I was in remission within that six-month period. Of course this does not happen with every patient, but it is worth keeping abreast of the latest advances in determining treatment particular to individual cancers.

New technologies, approaches, and pharmaceuticals are made available with each passing day. It is worth asking around to try and find those that fit your unique situation. This tip saved my life once. May it do the same for you!

15.

You Can't Call It a Wooden Stool

MAKING TOUGH DECISIONS

Master Baizhang challenged two students to a Zen duel by
pointing to a water pitcher and posing the following ques-
tion: "Without saying it's a water pitcher, what is it?"
Hua, the hotshot head monk said, "You can't call it
a wooden stool."
Then, out of nowhere, Ling You, the "lowly cook,"
kicked the pitcher over and left.

CAN YOU GUESS who the master picked as the winner? That's right, the cook won that duel fair and square. Why did the cook win? Because he got outside of preconceived ways of responding, to answer the challenge with spontaneous creativity. Hua, on the other hand, gave a carefully thought out, logical response, in line with what he had been taught to think. It was not a valid response to a Zen challenge.

Pure awareness, our true nature, transcends rational thought. Pure awareness is completely natural and is demonstrated naturally, unencumbered by effort, force, or rationalizing. Our rational minds are frequently the culprit in our own misery, after all. Zen cultivation helps us to get outside of the box of our own limiting preconceptions. We could all probably use such an authentic approach right about now.

The cook didn't turn away from or deny what he saw—he simply thought outside the box. A water pitcher is just something we call "water pitcher" when we see that it holds and pours water. There is no such object as a "water pitcher" until we have labeled it as such. The master wasn't challenging what a water pitcher is; he was challenging the students to reach beyond its mere label, to respond in a fresh and innovative way that transcends the act of labeling altogether.

Zen pushes us to see things for what they are: interdependent, coarising phenomena, rather than discrete entities with special labels. Master Baizhang did not want to hear certain words; he wanted a creative and spontaneous response to emerge from his students' true nature. These types of responses to life subvert our personal fears and self-doubts, allowing us to feel and behave in accord with our nature, without artifice.

What we perceive with the five senses through the filter of our preconceptions is not reality. We often get stuck on a specific perception of things, which then determines how we react to them. If we perceive something as overwhelming or scary, then it is for us in reality overwhelming and scary. To someone else, though, it may be neither overwhelming nor scary. In other words, if we can change the way we look at things, we can change our reality.

The cook showed no fear or worry about breaking a perfectly good water pitcher. He was able to see beyond "water pitcher, and respond appropriately to the challenge. That alone is a great lesson. We can all benefit from responding to life's challenges like that cook. He showed us what it looks like to take action without letting self-doubt and personal fear get in the way. Certainly there are places in your life where this might be helpful. If you change how you approach something you find difficult, if you can take away the "difficult" label and see it for what it is, it becomes easier.

If there is something you are afraid to look at, or afraid to do, take the time to get outside of the perspective of fear:

- Slow your body and mind down. Sit quietly and let yourself breathe naturally.
- Focus on the slow, deep inhalation and exhalation of breath. Feel your whole body relax.
- Picture yourself transcending fear or worry, stepping free from preconceptions with both eyes wide open.
- Let go of the label you've given the situation and try to see it for what it is: just another thing.

If you have been putting something off that needs doing—perhaps you soon have a treatment of some kind that you've been afraid of—take the time and space to go beyond your rational mind and find that fearless, spontaneous space where there are no labels, and from which you can act decisively, powerfully, or even humorously. I am sure that you can. We all have it in us. If a "lowly cook" can do it, so can you.

A fresh perspective yields a fresh response.

16.

When the Moon Reaches
the Window

SETTING SIMPLE GOALS

A boastful monk once told Zen Master Zhaozhou that
he read from seven to ten sutras per day.
The monk asked Old Zhao how many sutras
he read per day.
Old Zhao replied, "A word a day."

THE MASTER reminds us that little steps still take us
where we want to go. It may have taken him longer to
get there, but think of how much more he was able to
savor each step. He also reminds us of the benefit of setting simple goals.

When you set a simple goal, you have a greater likeli-
hood of meeting it. We all need something to look forward
to, and we all have things that we need to get done. The
first few steps are key. Why not keep them small'n'sweet?

Hardcore Zen practitioners were known to meditate
until the "moon reaches the window"—that is, until night
comes—and only then to call it quits for the day. That is

an example of a big step. While it is impressive to meditate all day, we may find that we have plenty of other, more realistic and achievable goals to reach.

An example of a simple step is to say that on days when you are tired, you will get in bed to begin the evening's rest when the moon reaches the window. Or perhaps you'll get the ever-growing pile of dishes done before the moon reaches the window.

- If you journal (or want to), try to journal a sentence a day.
- You might even try condensing the day into just once sentence, one phrase, or even one word.
- Read an inspirational quote a day to help put you in the right frame of mind.
- If you want to exercise, take one walk a day, regardless of the length.
- Or respond to an email a day.

So what's today's activity? Begin where you are—but begin!

17.
The Ultimate Teaching

REMEMBERING WHAT MATTERS

Monk: "What is the ultimate teaching of all buddhas?"
Master Fayan: "You too have it."

THE ULTIMATE TEACHING is clear: you already have everything you need. You are already complete, whole, and an integral part of existence. Master Linji taught that the only thing that gets in the way of living this reality is our lack of faith in ourselves. He strongly encouraged us to stop searching for the answers outside and instead to turn our awareness inward.

Almost every tip in this book comes from this awakened view. What we think, say, and do matters. Why? Because our words and actions reflect our peace of mind—or lack thereof. The effects of our cultivation of peace of mind ripple out into the world around us. This is basic behavioral science. Regardless of one's diagnosis or prognosis, the world can certainly use more words and actions arising from peace of mind rather than from fear or a lack of faith in oneself.

While we may already have everything we need to cultivate a more awakened view, we are constantly faced with challenges. The masters encourage us to cultivate and maintain an awakened view through it all—the good, the bad, and the ugly. This is of course harder than it sounds, which is why we call Zen a "practice"!

Bring an enhanced sense of presence and awareness to a small part of your day in a way that will help you respond positively and beneficially despite any hardship.

- Say a silent, personal healing prayer when you take your pills or when you sit down to a meal.
- Make a mindful effort to be more present during your daily exercise routine.
- Practice deep and relaxing breathing when waiting in line.
- When your visitors leave you, cultivate a sense of gratefulness for their care.
- Send some healing energy to yourself when you get in bed each night: One way of doing this is to place your hands over the area where your cancer is, and visualize, as you breathe, an alchemical fire coming from your hands and melting the cancer away for good.
- Or place one hand over the center of your chest and one just below your belly button. Visualize white, healing energy coming into your body from your hands. See it energize and fill your whole body, stim-

ulating your immune system and increasing your body's energy levels. There are many ways to do this, and you can even invent your own. The important thing is to do it with a sense of genuine self-care.

They say that to test precious jade, it must be passed through fire. When you feel the heat, remember that you can choose a different, a more awakened response to your situation. No matter how difficult things may get, it is important not to lose sight of what matters—our actions toward others and ourselves. You, too, have the capacity to benefit the world. Don't forget it.

II.
Soothing Your Spirit

18.

Tree Stumps

DEVELOPING A MEDITATION PRACTICE

*Master Shishuang's disciples were called "tree stumps"
because they were known to sit in meditation so long
that they resembled tree stumps. Master Yantou spoke
up in favor of the happy medium. He said, "If you spend
all of your time sitting in meditation like a clay statue
in someone's home, you are not being very useful!"*

HE'S RIGHT—we all have obligations that we need to
meet, people to help, and things to do in the world. Who
wants to be a clay statue or a tree stump anyway? Many
of us turn to meditation practice after the shit has hit the
fan. Others have had a long-standing desire to learn how
to meditate, but have felt intimidated for one reason or
another. We don't need to be bald monks in a monastery
to meditate in a meaningful way.

The secret to meditation is very simple: do it. How,
when, where, and for how long are just details, all of
which can be adjusted to fit your life. Have just five minutes at work? Great! Close your door, set aside whatever

you are working on, and meditate. Have thirty minutes? Great! Meditate.

In Zen we begin to learn how to meditate using a one-through-ten counting meditation. Zen meditation, or *zazen*, is a form of concentration meditation. Concentrating on numbers is a great, challenging way to begin to quiet and focus our monkey minds. If you have five minutes you can practice it.

- Sit with a straight spine and rest your palms on your thighs.
- Keep your eyes slightly open, with a soft gaze on the floor ahead of you.
- As you inhale, think the number "one" (say it silently to yourself inside your mind).
- As you exhale, repeat "one" in your mind.
- As you inhale again, switch your focus to the number "two," and then repeat "two" silently, in your mind as you exhale.
- Continue in this way, working your way up to ten. If and when you reach ten, begin again at one.
- If your mind wanders, start back at one.
- Repeat the sequence until you feel the session should end.

It takes most people a while to be able to count to ten without their mind wandering off. This is perfectly normal. The key is to bring your mind back to "one" whenever you notice that you've stopped counting. Even though you may find this to be tougher than it sounds, you will feel the benefits of a still mind relatively quickly. The more regularly you practice, the easier it will be.

19.

Meditation in Action

BRINGING PRESENCE INTO YOUR DAY

You can meditate for many years and still be a jackass.

PERHAPS YOU'VE SEEN THIS; maybe you've been spared. Zen Master Hakuin used to say that meditation in action is thousands of times superior to meditation in stillness. In other words, it is what happens after you get up off the cushion or chair that matters most.

Meditation is not defined by placing your bottom on a fancy cushion, and it certainly does not mean sitting still and spacing out. Meditation is a state of mind, a practice of concentration or awareness. Wouldn't it be more useful to be able to remain calm, present, and aware throughout the day, rather than just for the fifteen to thirty minutes we spend on the cushion?

How can we meditate while engaging in day-to-day activities? Start here:

- Bring your attention to your breath.
- Feel the air coming in and out of your nostrils.

- Feel how breathing moves and relaxes different parts of your body.
- Relax your body deeper with each breath.
- Practice this for a while.

Once we are able to keep our mental focus on the breath, we are ready to bring meditation into action:

- Bring your awareness to the breath and feel your body relax, as above.
- Maintain awareness of the breath as you get up to do something active.
- Begin by maintaining awareness of the breath and the body as you make a cup of tea, do a few stretches, or wash the dishes.
- When you notice your mind has wandered, bring it back to your breath and carry on. See how long you can keep part of your conscious awareness on the act of breathing as you engage in routine activities.

The secret to this practice is that we must stay present and focused in order to remember our breath. As you practice, your ability to remain calm and present will strengthen, and this strength can be used at will.

20.

Make Every Place a Temple

CREATING A HOME ALTAR

Old Master Zhao once said:
"A furnace destroys a metal buddha,
a fire destroys a wooden buddha,
water destroys a mud buddha,
but the genuine buddha resides within you."

MASTER ZHAO realized that what is truly sacred lies within us and cannot be destroyed. We are an essential part of the sacred.

Many of us go to church, to temple, or to some other place where spiritual and religious folks gather to meet friends and recharge our spiritual batteries for the week. Some of us may prefer to fly solo, finding sustenance in spiritual literature or the occasional workshop or class. Whatever the case may be, the cancer journey can disrupt our normal pattern of rejuvenating ourselves with such visits. Master Zhao's realization reminds us that we can make any place sacred. We too can visit a sacred space without leaving the comforts of our own homes.

Home altars are common in Asian households. You have probably seen one in an Asian-American-owned business. A small home altar allows us to bring sacred space into our homes and can be very useful when we don't feel up to getting dressed up and venturing out. Of course, practicing with other likeminded people can be very uplifting, but sometimes it just isn't going to happen, for whatever reason.

You can find fancy, traditional home altars online, but you don't have to spend a penny to create your own altar. A home altar is really just a small place in the house that is set aside and arranged in a way that helps bring us in touch with what we find deep, enduring, and meaningful— things that bring out what is sacred within us.

We can transform a space in our homes as small as a shelf or a part of a desk or table into an altar.

- Set up your altar as a small space that engages all of your senses in whatever ways seem most pleasing to you. For example, put a picture of someone or something you find spiritually inspiring, such as a special place in nature, your friends or family, or a spiritual teacher of some sort in a prominent place on your altar. Add something nice on the eyes like flowers, a small statue or icon, or a candle. Find the perfect (or perfect enough) incense holder and some incense you like so that you can have a formal incense-lighting ritual and make things smell pretty.

- I like to keep a small metal singing bowl with a striker on my altar, and I ring it to begin and end meditation sessions. A small bell or crystal bowl also works well for this purpose. If your place can get a little chilly, you can keep a comfy shawl or warm scarf near your altar to keep you wrapped and warm during meditation or contemplation, or when you choose to read something inspiring nearby.

- Some people like to put fruit such as oranges or fresh strawberries on the altar. They can be there as an offering, or just for color, but we can eat the fruit to stimulate our sense of taste after meditation. I love this idea, as your senses are usually heightened after a good sit.

You can sit before your altar to pray, meditate, journal, read, or to just stare into space when you need to.

A small home altar can help us remember that our temple is always here within us, wherever we are. We can touch our spirits and recharge our batteries anywhere. Making an ordinary space extraordinary is a way to celebrate the spiritual at home.

And you will have a special spot just for you.

21.
Be a Light unto Yourself

SLOWING DOWN AND CHECKING IN

When Buddha was at the very end of his life,
    his students expressed sadness and fear that they
    would be unable to deepen their spiritual understanding
    or experience awakening without the Buddha's presence.
    They said to Buddha that he was their light, and because
    he was leaving, darkness was descending upon them.
Buddha's last words to his disciples were,
    "Be a light unto yourself."

THIS QUOTE from the Buddha is often found in Zen meditation halls or *zendos*. We may also translate it as "Turn the light inward on your self nature."

The answers to our deepest spiritual questions cannot be found outside of ourselves. No one else can show us who we truly are. Teachers and their teachings are like a finger pointing at the moon: they can help to guide us, but they are not themselves what we are being guided to. A finger is not the moon, and staring at a pointing finger will not get us to the moon.

From the Zen point of view we are all interconnected and interdependent. We are each an essential part of the whole. In that sense, we are not really set apart from everything. Everything is reflected within us, and we are reflected within it. The only way to answer the spiritual questions we carry is to turn our attention from the finger outside of ourselves toward what lies within us. We must slow down and look into ourselves.

Take the time to shine a light into the corners of your mind and spirit. Light chases away darkness and shadows.

- Amazing things happen when you take time to slow down and check in with yourself. How have you really been doing? Face it and get over yourself.
- Take a moment in silence and stillness to turn your light inward and look within.
- Within this silent space, listen to what you need from yourself to help you feel better right now. For many of us, it begins with a shift in thinking or attitude.
- Remind yourself of what is available to you right here in your life.
- Remind yourself of your amazing and numerous positive attributes.
- Review your recent or past actions that have helped or benefitted others. These kindnesses matter and ripple out into the world. Really allow yourself to feel this truth.

Once you shine the light on your thoughts and actions, continue to turn your light toward the places where forgiveness can serve you by freeing up some headspace and breathing room within.

- Breathe deeply and relax your body and mind.
- With each out breath practice letting go of tension and forgiving perceived wrongs.
- Let go just a little bit more with each subsequent breath. This could take some time, so give yourself all the time and space you need to accomplish this worthy task.
- Continue letting go of anger or other tense emotions with each breath.
- When you feel the session should end, wind it up with a bit of gratitude: think of the many little things (or one big thing) for which you are grateful.
- Let that feeling of gratitude overflow and fill your whole body.
- When you leave your session, carry this abundant and glowing gratitude with you.

Shine your light brightly and often. Allowing no corners of your mind to remain dark is absolutely enlightening!

22.

The Sound of One Hand Clapping

LISTENING MEDITATION

Listen!
   Right now. Just purely listen to your surroundings
   for a moment or two.
What do you hear?

IN ORDER TO truly listen, we must slow down. Slowing down is by definition good when you have cancer, and even when you don't. Zen teaches us to slow down until we not only hear sounds, we see, taste, smell, and feel them. Meditation practice allows us to experience ourselves as the sound itself.

You may have heard the Zen koan "What is the sound of one hand clapping?" The true sound of one hand clapping cannot be described in words. It is an experience. We only experience sound in that way when we slow down and listen with all of our senses. Rarely do we slow down enough to listen with our whole being—where we pay total and perfect attention to the sound around us at any particular moment. Even when music is playing, we rarely stop everything we are doing to take it in fully and completely.

Sound and music can be transcendent, eye opening, and healing. We all know that sound can have soothing, therapeutic properties. Daoist shamans and masters of Chinese medicine have used sound in their healing for centuries. Surely we all have experienced the rejuvenating uplift of a great song. We can meditate on the natural sounds around us, or even choose some music on which to meditate.

I used a guided visualization CD almost every time I had a marathon chemo day. I began the disc when the chemo began. Guided visualization helped me to relax, took me on a nice journey, and made me feel powerful, strong, healthy, and vibrant. It was like a minivacation. Sometimes I would follow it up with some music to keep the good vibes going. The art of deep listening opens us up to "meditative mind," where we are no longer off in our thoughts, but instead we become one with the object of our listening.

- Try scheduling a specific time during your day or during the week when you put on a piece of music that touches you or takes you away to another time or place.
- If you have headphones, use them.
- Sit or lie down, close your eyes, and let the music take you on an inner journey.

- Allow yourself to become fully absorbed in the sounds of the music.
- Afterward, you'll likely notice a nice shift in your psyche and spirit.

The key is to discover what works best for you. Some will prefer nature sounds, affirmations, or a special genre of music rather than guided imagery. Find what soothes your soul and crank it up. Learn which pieces of music or guided meditation recordings help turn down the internal noise and turn up the calm.

That is the sound of one hand clapping.

23.

The Mind Is an Unruly Monkey

STILLING THE MIND

In Chinese Zen, they use the term "monkeymind" to describe when our minds jump from thought to thought like a monkey through the trees.

"Monkeymind" is an apt metaphor for our everyday chatty, wandering, thinking minds. Imagine five minutes of inner thoughts captured on tape. The sheer volume of thoughts that occur in that short span, not to mention their randomness, is astounding. We all have an experience like this when we begin to pay attention to our minds.

We are exposed to enormous amounts of information and mental stimulation all day long. Computers, cell phones, television, gadgets and gizmos—there is plenty to be distracted by, and our monkeyminds feed on such distractions. I should note that this condition did not begin with technology, as the term monkeymind comes from ancient times in China, before they even had electricity. Relationship issues, family issues, money issues, and job issues are all fabulous mental distractions, each of which alone is enough to set our minds off and running, not to mention what a combination of these can do!

Our brains and nervous systems need to periodically rest and reboot. At some point, we all need to slow down and come to stillness. Imagine stirred up, muddy water. As it becomes still again, the dirt settles to the bottom, and the water becomes clear. Zen asks us, "Can you still your mind until it is clear like water or blank like a white silk canvas?"

The answer is "yes," but it's actually pretty tough to do. That's why we call Zen a "practice." When we first begin Zen meditation, we are often instructed to count from one to ten in our heads. This technique forces us to focus our minds on a single task. This focus helps to slow internal chatter way down. In this exercise, you will count as your chest expands as you inhale and contracts as you exhale. If we practice this counting technique regularly, we begin notice a newfound stillness that deeply relaxes both our bodies and minds.

- To begin, find a comfortable position. I recommend a seated position, as it is easy to fall asleep when lying down. Sit with your spine upright. If you are in a chair, you can rest your back on the back of your chair and allow your feet to be flat on the ground. Or you can try sitting on a meditation cushion with your legs folded in any position that is comfortable for you. Allow your hands to rest palms up in your lap on the upper part of your legs.

- Breathe slowly, deeply, and comfortably, without forcing it.
- Count to four in your head as you inhale fully and deeply and fill your lungs from the bottoms to the tops.
- Exhale as slowly as is comfortable without forcing it. Try to stretch the out breath about twice as long, to a count of eight if you can.
- Periodically check in and release any tension in your body.
- Repeat for as long as you wish.

The more single-minded focus you bring to counting the beats of each breath, the more tension you will feel released from your nervous system.

24.

Donkey Milk

LOOKING FOR SPIRITUAL TEACHERS

*Master Guishan said, "A single drop of milk from
real teachers and their disciples is more valuable
than six ladles of donkey milk."*

IN OTHER WORDS, a drop of profound truth is worth many
swigs of lesser—or even worse, misleading—information.

So where are the real teachers? How can we find the
truth? Most of the time, we have to drink a lot of donkey
milk before we find the pure taste we've been seeking. In
the old days, you would have to journey hundreds or even
thousands of miles to find a good teacher. Now it can be
as easy as sitting in front of your computer, or picking up
a book. How do we choose a good teacher?

- First, go with your gut.
- Who have you come across that interests, challenges,
  and inspires you?
- If no one comes to mind, get recommendations from
  friends.

- The Internet is a great place to find videos or recordings of teachers working in the world today. A simple Internet search using words you are interested in, such as "Buddhism and compassion," or "Zen and mindfulness," or even "dharma talk on self-love," can lead you on the right path.

- There are also many bookstores out there with sections on spirituality. Perhaps there is one near you that you haven't yet visited, or haven't visited in a while. This is a perfect excuse for an outing. Take your time to look through the shelves and see if any books jump out at you. You can even ask someone who works in that section to give you recommendations and to let you know what is popular.

- Explore what different teachers have to say, and how what they say speaks to you. If someone floats your boat, look for a nearby workshop by that person or by one of her students. Of course the best situation would be to have in-person experiences with people who inspire you.

So how do you know if a teacher is any good or if she is just doling out donkey milk? Here are a few tips. First, beware of teachers who talk only about themselves. It is one thing to share one's experiences and feelings in order to clarify a point or get a message across; it is another to spend an entire talk on "me, me, me." If someone's talk is riddled with "me's" and "I's," I have often found that the talk rarely goes deep or leaves one with much food for thought.

My suspicion is often raised when a teacher charges an exorbitant fee to hear him speak, especially when it is paired with claims that he can perform "healing miracles." If a teacher is in it for the healing and to empower others, he almost always charges a reasonable fee, and he won't make grandiose claims without the ability to back them with irrefutable proof (his own stories and recollections do not constitute "irrefutable proof"). You may have things like this that raise your hackles too. Trust your intuition and go with your gut. If what someone says or claims seems too good to be true, chances are it is.

Sometimes it takes just a few words said in a new way to change how we've been thinking or feeling. Anyone and anything can be a true teacher, if we let them be. A quote read at the perfect moment or the sound of a baby laughing can open our eyes to profound truths, given the right mindset.

In Zen, a superb teacher is said to teach by "transmission," which is the ability to transmit wisdom, knowledge, and the "state of awakened mind" simply by the way she is in the world. These types of teachers are the real gems, and they are not just found in Zen circles. Their actions speak louder than their words, and their actions are also in accord with their words.

Remember, you need not take the word "teacher" so literally. Any experience and anyone can be a teacher. For a long time, my greatest teachers were Japanese haiku poets and Chinese poets from the Tang Dynasty. These poets spoke directly to my heart and enriched my spirit in a way no living teacher had. Nonetheless, I continued my search for a living teacher with whom I felt some kind of connection or bond, and I finally found him.

Become a seeker so that you can become a finder! There is no need to drink donkey milk, as there is plenty of milk from real teachers out there to be found.

25.

The Summit Is Obscured

CULTIVATING MOMENTS OF AWARENESS

A skeptic asked the famous Zen Master Moshan,
  "What is Moshan?"
She replied, "It's peak cannot be seen."

SHE WAS VERY CLEVER; her name was Chinese for Mo Mountain. The master means that we cannot see, or even describe with words, who we truly are. This is comforting news, despite what we may think. If we spend all of our time looking for answers, we risk missing what is right here in front of us now. There will always be questions for which we have no answers. With this in mind, let's rest a bit to give our searching brains and strained nerves a little break.

Have you taken a good breath today? Have you paid attention to your body today? Have you heard what it's telling you? Have you heard any birds singing today? Let's stop and tend to what's going on in this very moment.

This very moment is the only time you can rest and heal. Take a break from your to-do list. Let a few summits remain obscured for just a short while longer. Balance active moments with moments of stillness.

- Completely relax your body.
- Let your thoughts slow down so you can hear any messages your intuition or body is trying to share.
- Listen to the environment around you without trying to do anything.
- Slow all parts of you down . . . way, way, way down.

Carve out a regular pocket of time in which you can just chill out. Use this time to tune in to what is in front of you, or better yet, to tune in to what's inside of you. Don't worry about what to do next. Your nervous system will certainly thank you for the stillness.

When we practice this type of presence or awareness— replacing doing with being—we begin to experience a sense of deep relaxation within minutes. Stillness is an efficient gateway to your deeper self. Master Moshan spent much of her life in stillness, and she gained tremendous clarity and wisdom. This is the surest way to get in touch with your deeper self and real needs.

When you can be still like a mountain, check in with yourself and just be. Take a break from all the doing. When your heart and mind are as still as a mountain, you realize that you are spirit, divine—a buddha—having a human experience.

"You are the biggest mystery," said Master Touzi.
And, boy, wasn't he right?

26.

Sit in the Bodhi Seat

OWNING YOUR POWER

Junpo Roshi frequently—and lovingly—shouts
at us students, "Take your seat!"

WHAT SEAT is he talking about? The seat that is your birthright. The seat of awakened mind, also called the Bodhi Seat. "Bodhi" means awakened mind or the awakened state.

Junpo Roshi believes that only you can empower you. "This seat will not be given to you! You must take it!" he exhorts.

When the going gets rough, it may be time to get going—to change things up and take hold of our seat. The only way to do that is to tap into the inherent power of who we are. When we truly take our seat, our view expands in new and often unpredictable ways. We are honest with ourselves and act with integrity.

What is this seat like? Master Mazu said it was peace. Sure, it is peaceful. But it is also a place of fierce, wise, and compassionate presence. Fierce, wise, and compassionate—three of our best qualities.

What does "taking your seat" mean? It means dropping into the truth of who we are and taking a fresh look, free from our usual judgments and worries. We can see things newly from the awakened mind, the mind beyond the fears of our egos: bigger mind, collective mind, connected mind. From here we see a bigger, more accurate picture of who we are.

Now that you know that you can take your seat, the question is, "Will you?" Remember, no one will give it to you; only you can take your seat. You alone must choose to use your innate greater perspective. Are you willing to open your mind to your own truths? Try on this type of presence right now.

- Begin on the inside to start. Take this moment in silence and stillness and think about what step or steps you can take to do something that benefits your mind, body, or spirit.
- To be "fiercely compassionate" is to have the kind of compassion that doesn't allow for excuses and ways out of doing what is most beneficial for yourself and others. Fierce compassion drives us to take responsibility for our thoughts and actions and admit that we are the bosses of our own lives. No one else is in the driver's seat. Yes, there may be little in life we

have control over, but only we can control our own thoughts and actions. If we don't, who does?

- Fierce compassion makes us take an honest look at what needs to be done, and then do it. No excuses, no laziness. This how we gain wisdom. We gain a little more wisdom each time we exercise our ability to take care of ourselves in ways that may not be particularly easy for us.

When you take your Bodhi Seat, your natural inner strength and peace will reveal themselves.

27.

Light Another's Lamp
and Your Own Path Brightens

BEING OF SERVICE

*When Zen wisdom is transmitted, it is referred to
as a transmission of "the lamp."*

"The lamp" is the light of Zen wisdom and compassion.
The candle in one lamp can light innumerable other
lamps and still not be diminished. Likewise, when you
light another person's lamp, the path becomes brighter
for the both of you.

Want to know the secret to getting out of a funk? Do
something for someone else. Yes, this even applies to
those of us who are in need ourselves. The truth is that
we are all in need in some way or another!

Everyone knows it is good karma to help others. Plus,
focusing on someone else can help to get us out of our
own drama and into the world around us. Certainly we all
have some talent or skill that a friend or stranger would
appreciate. You might be a good cook, or a gifted gardener.

When I don't feel like going out, I like to have people

over for a meal, or prepare an informal tea ceremony for a friend or two. Helping others can be as simple as writing a small recurring check to a charity, or having a fixed monthly donation automatically charged to your bank or credit card if you have the wherewithal. Many local public radio stations offer this option. The Internet is overflowing with out-of-the-box ideas for giving. No gesture is too small; it just needs to be big enough to allow us to focus on something or someone besides ourselves for a bit.

In Buddhism it is said that true happiness comes not from thinking about one's self but from thinking about others. Focusing on the needs of others and letting go of our own drama relieves our own suffering by helping us release self-clinging, ego attachment, and the feeling that we are the only ones with "real problems." The truth is that we are all in the same soup. All around the world humans suffer from the same wide variety of problems.

Being human means that we will experience suffering from time to time. When we turn our hearts toward others, even in some small way, we feel a sense of connectedness, a sense of being "one with" that is often missing when we get stuck in our own dramas. We receive as much as or even more than we give. We receive it in the form of feeling good about our actions, feeling like we can and have made a difference; feeling the reality that the world benefits from each and every small act of kindness.

It is easy for your whole world to revolve around having cancer. On occasion, that may even be necessary. Still, when you take the time to do something positive for another, whether it is a human, an animal, the environment, or whatever cause you champion, you will always feel better.

When you brighten someone else's day, your day brightens too. Bring more light into the world for yourself and others. Brighten the path for us all!

28.

Riding an Ox
While in Search of an Ox

RECOGNIZING YOUR TRUE NATURE

*When Master Baizhang heard one of his students
complain that he felt something was missing, he scolded
him, saying, "You are riding an ox in search of an ox."*

HUH?

Zen masters speak in riddles to provoke thought or,
rather, to provoke a state beyond thought. The master is
pointing out that we already have what we are seeking,
and that we are even using it to seek. Here, the ox is our
true nature, the truth of who we are in essence. No part
of our true nature can ever be lost. The truth of who we
are is always right here, changelessly enduring each and
every adventure and misadventure that life brings.

There are times when you may feel as if you've lost
something after being diagnosed with cancer. You may
feel like you've lost your vitality, or your peace of mind,
or even your sense of self. It may be hard to know where
to look to find what you feel is missing.

But Zen masters know just where to start. You can only be whole; no diagnosis can take away your wholeness. There is no need to search outside for who you are. Not only is there no need; what you seek cannot be found there. You have more important things to do with your time than to seek something that can never be lost! What we may lose is our perspective, or our connection to the deepest part of who we are. The Zen approach is to turn our gaze inward, where we discover everything, and nothing can be lost.

Many years ago, one of my cancer patients, Alejandro, had lost the meaning of his life after years of living with cancer. I didn't know what to do for him at that point, so I did an I-Ching reading to get some new direction or insight into how I might be able to help him. The reading essentially said that I should focus on the past, which was a nice starting point for my next visit. Instead of giving him a treatment that day, I asked if he had any old photos around (I was coming to his home at that point). He said he did, and we looked through photos from when he was in his twenties and thirties—photos from all different parts of his life. When we were through, with tears in his eyes he said, "You know, I've really done so many special things with my life." He was able to feel and remember that his life mattered; that what he had done mattered. I consider that the best "treatment" I've ever given.

- Take some time to reconnect with yourself. Revisit the memories and experiences that you've accumulated in life and which make you who you are.
- Look back through photo albums to catch a glimpse of yourself in the making.
- Review things you've created in life—maybe photos, drawings, songs, or writing.Invite a long-time friend to sit and reminisce about the life you've shared.
- Take the time to remember the contributions you've made to those around you, and to think of all the people whose lives you've touched.
- It doesn't take much to spark memories of times when you felt completely "you."

The meaning of our lives is expressed in what we do (and do not do) with the time we are given. Take a few moments today to reconnect with the parts of yourself that you may have neglected, but which are nonetheless lying dormant within you. Bring those parts out to play and remember that you cannot be anything but whole. You can only be wholly you.

When we lose touch with ourselves we forget our wholeness and end up searching for it, riding an ox in search of an ox. Why spend time looking for something you already have? It is simply a matter of recognizing and returning to yourself.

29.
No Self, No Other

OPENING TO INTERCONNECTION

A Zen master nicknamed "Tiger" said,
"There isn't one being that isn't you."

WE ALL SUFFER at some point. It is inevitable. We all take turns, it seems, and we all respond to suffering differently. But we are all in the same soup.

As a Chinese medicine doctor whose job it was to help keep people healthy, becoming a cancer patient was especially humbling and confusing. Cancer was supposed to happen to "other people," who didn't take good enough care of themselves. I used to think that. Luckily, reality has since disabused me of this sort of ridiculous thought. How we respond to life's challenges is up to us. Sometimes it helps to acknowledge that we are not the first ones to be diagnosed with cancer; we are not alone. Cancer diagnoses are actually a common, daily occurrence.

Think about that.

There is nothing extraordinary or unusual about being diagnosed with cancer. It is unfortunate, but true. Cancer simply is what it is, and we are a part of it. The practice of Zen can help us to recognize the extent of our interconnectedness and interdependence in the web of life. Seeing less and less difference between self and other, we begin to have greater compassion for others and greater compassion for ourselves.

It may appear to us that everything and everyone is discreet and distinct from one another. Zen challenges this view. From a Zen perspective, we only see things as distinct entities because we have been conditioned to by our own special and distinct sense of "I." Flowing out of this sense of "I" comes an illusory sense of isolation from others and from the world in which we find ourselves. For me, it took a cancer diagnosis to wake up to the greater, more inclusive, less judgmental reality, and I already thought I was there!

We have all been conditioned to feel like discrete ego entities, despite the deeper, preconditioned reality that we are inextricably a part of the whole; the entire cosmos. We cannot be separated from this whole, because we are this whole. The Zen view of reality holds that for any one thing to exist, it must be dependent on, and interconnect with, something else. This is traditionally called "dependent coarising," but Thich Nhat Hanh calls it "interbeing." You wouldn't and couldn't exist without your parents, the sun, the rain, the earth, and on and on it goes.

Japanese Zen master Dogen once said, "When one side is illuminated, the other side remains in darkness." In other words, for there to be a yin, there must be a yang. If you only see one side, you miss the other side. If you only see one side, you miss the totality. Likewise, for there to be an ego, there must also be a Buddha nature—a quality of mind in which the perception of difference is unified. If we only see ego, we miss our Buddha nature. When we tap into our Buddha nature, we become intimately aware of our interconnection with others.

These are fabulous concepts to contemplate and discuss, but they are a hell of a lot more powerful and life altering when their truth is experienced firsthand. Cultivating a practice of meditation allows us to recognize the truth of our situation more easily. Like any art, learning to see the world differently can take time, but most cities have at least a few Buddhist centers where regular meditation classes are held and where one can seek out training in the art of meditation with an experienced teacher.

Experiential understanding of the nonduality of interbeing may also be gained through koan practice. Responding to a koan requires that we bypass ordinary intellectual tools such as logic and reason, in order to tap into a knowledge that is deeper than egotistic mind. Koan practice also requires the dynamic guidance of an experienced teacher capable of testing your understanding and pushing you in directions you may not have seen yourself. As with meditation, a quick Internet search will lead you to local circles of Zen people who work with koans.

My cancer diagnosis really brought home the reality—

not just the philosophical notion—that all of my patients, and all of humanity, were the same as me. As a result of it, my practice of meditation and work with koans deepened. Now the truth of interbeing seems crystal clear to me. Of course I will always see "self and other" and "this and that," but the superficiality of these seems much more apparent than it did before cancer, and the deeper reality shines through more readily.

It is my sincere hope that this brief reflection will motivate you to explore the deeper reality through meditation or whichever spiritual practice appeals to you. Then, if we were to meet and embrace, there would be no one hugging and no one being hugged, only the warm embrace of what is.

30.

Your Treasure Is Within, Containing All You Need

REMEMBERING WHO YOU ARE

Master Huihai wisely said,
"Your treasure is within, containing all you need."

I TURN TO HIS warm words when I am not looking quite as lovely as I would like to on the outside. Some days I would see myself and think "Mirror, Mirror, on the wall . . . who the hell is that staring back at me?!"

There are side effects to almost every type of cancer treatment. This is true even of some of the more natural approaches. A lovely rash turned me purple, dotting me with hundreds of tiny white pimple-things from the crown of my head to just below my chest and mid-back. It went on for months, affording me ample opportunity to display this sexy look over and over in a wide variety of settings. I haven't gone bald yet, despite the predictions, but I have a mantra prepared for that eventuality: Bald is Buddhaful! Feel free to use it.

These days when I look in a mirror, I hardly recognize the person standing before me. At times like these it is nice to remember that my true treasure, my essence, resides deep within me, unaffected by any and all side effects known to humanity.

Your true treasure abides, too.

This part of you, the deepest truth of who you are, has nothing to do with your physical appearance. It remains unchanged no matter how funky you may come to look. You know who you are inside. You are still the same book, the same unfolding life story, but now you have a new, more interesting cover.

Of course, there are little steps we can take to help ourselves feel more comfortable in public. Take them. That being said, it is essential to remember that there is nothing to search for outside of ourselves. At our core, we are connected to everyone and everything around us, with nothing left out. We have all we need to make it through. Now is the perfect time to practice making contact with that essential part of yourself, that handsome or beautiful person inside, watching and witnessing what is unfolding outside. Here's how to take an honest look and find out what your true self needs to feel more like the gem you are. You'll find that whatever it is, it is already and always within reach.

- This exercise is most easily practiced sitting down, preferably at a table or desk, so you can take your sweet time.

- Bring a mirror. A tabletop mirror is best, but a hand-held mirror is a close second. If you have neither, you can of course practice this in front of any kind of mirror you happen to have.

- Position a chair in front of a mirror so that you can see your entire face and head. Your face and head should take up most of the mirror, if possible.

- Begin by taking a good, thorough look at your appearance. Try to do so without any judgment, but if judgments or feelings arise, just let them happen without attaching to them.

- Let any feelings or judgments come and go as you focus your awareness on your outward appearance. Take as long as feels right. Whatever emotions arise, acknowledge them and allow them to pass through you. (This is a great practice in itself.)

- When you feel ready, bring your focus to the reflection of your eyes only. The eyes are the windows to the soul, and in Chinese medicine, we say that they are a reflection of your *shen*, or spirit. Look right into your own eyes and visualize connecting to the part of you that is responsible for seeing; the part of you that animates all of your body's functions.

- Now ask yourself the question, "Who is seeing?" Your eyes could not see without this "who." The who that is seeing is always inside your physical form, regardless of the changing nature of that form. The

who is most definitely not your physical form. Try
to answer the question: Who is seeing?

- Connect with that "who" with love, respect, and
appreciation. That unchanging "who" is the truth
of who you are, regardless of your appearance. Allow
these feelings of love, respect, and appreciation to
wash through your whole being. Take as long as you
wish to feel and experience these feelings from your
inside, out.

Your true treasure is the answer to the question, "Who
is seeing?" Your true treasure is the amazing life-force
energy that animates your body and mind. This treasure
is there to help you get through whatever you need to get
through. When you take the time to acknowledge the part
of you that is not your body, the feelings of gratitude will
be bodily experienced and will benefit the body as well
as the mind.

Your true treasure has always been the seer, not the
seen.

31.
The Master's Special Medicine

APPRECIATING THE ORDINARY

A monk asked Master Xianglin,
"What is the master's special medicine?"
"It's none other than ordinary taste," the master replied.
"How about those who ingest it?" the monk asked.
"Why not taste it and see?"

THIS BRIEF EXCHANGE, which only appears to be about medicine, is a great demonstration of Zen in action. What is the master trying to teach the monk? The monk is looking for something special, something that perhaps only Master Xianglin can offer. The master makes it clear that his "special medicine" is nothing special. It is the ordinary that is special, and the ordinary is all that the master has to offer.

The monk continues, and surprisingly the master remains as patient as a grandmother. The monk asks about what happens to students who take the master's medicine. The monk is "talking about doing." This is a

Zen no-no. It is like talking about how to golf, rather than learning how to golf. If we were interested in mastering golf, which would we choose? Talking and doing are different. Shhh! Try it.

If we spend all of our time seeking something special, we overlook the value of the day-to-day goings on that comprise most of our lives. There are plenty of distractions pulling our attention toward what's new, bigger, and better. How about what is right under our noses? The ordinary is special, but we have to pay attention to notice.

The master encourages the monk to stop talking and to experience the master's teachings for himself. How can you experience these teachings for yourself? Paying single-minded attention to routine activities may appear easy, but we are so used to going throughout much of our day on autopilot that it usually takes some real effort to do this. It is best to begin right where you are. There is no need to find a special opportunity to practice mindfulness. When you add mindfulness to the mundane, you realize that even brushing your teeth is a kind of special medicine. Why? Because any practice of mindfulness brings a deeper appreciation of the extraordinariness of daily life.

A delightful way to begin a mindfulness practice is through mindful eating. The following is a great exercise to start you on your mindfulness path. Think of it as a little Zen starter practice.

- Choose a piece of fruit that you particularly love. If you can find an organic piece of fruit at the grocery store, choose that. Once you have your favorite fruit, bring it to the table and place it on a plate. (If you don't particularly enjoy fruit, find a type of fruit that you are okay with, just for this exercise. The exercise may change your mind!) Sit down with a knife next to your plate and nothing else on the table to distract you. Go as slowly and methodically as possible through each of the following steps. See if you can enjoy and savor the experience with each step.

- Begin by simply looking at the fruit. As you do so, clear your mind of all other thoughts and focus solely on the fruit.

- Observe and note its colors.

- Observe the textures.

- Is it hard, or does it give a little in your hand?

- Feel whether it is warm or cool or neutral in temperature.

- Bring your focus wholly to the fruit. When your mind wanders, bring it back to the fruit before you.

- Now smell the fruit. Does it have a smell? If not, and you have a knife, perhaps slice it and see if that releases an aroma. If slicing releases an aroma, note how it smells. Is it sweet-smelling? Sour-smelling? Does it make you salivate?

- Now close your eyes and take a bite or place a slice of the fruit in your mouth. Chew as slowly as you possibly can while enjoying and noticing the tastes and flavors released as you chew. It is very important to do this step very slowly so that you can experience the taste fully and completely.

- Continue to eat the whole fruit in the above manner. Notice if the flavor experience intensifies or lessens as you finish the whole fruit. Does the flavor linger in your mouth? If it does, does it change after a short while?

- To complete the exercise, with your eyes still closed, notice how your body feels after eating the fruit. Maybe you feel satisfied; maybe it made you hungrier. Do you have more energy, are you more calm than when you started, or perhaps both?

Find little ways to bring this single-minded focus into other parts of your day. Pay attention to what needs to be done and do it with mindfulness. Are you getting enough sleep? Bring the act of getting to bed early into your daily mindfulness routine. When the clock strikes 9 or 9:30 p.m., take a bath or get ready for bed. Notice each of your evening rituals and carry them out with your full attention.

Are you eating well? Notice what foods are missing from your diet, or whether you are skipping meals. Prepare a shopping list before you go shopping. Prepare your meals with your full attention, and when you eat, just eat.

Are you exercising? Take the time to figure out when

during each day you can add a mindful exercise routine, and then do it. When you exercise, bring your awareness to your breath and your body. Notice how you feel physically during and after a good walk, qigong, tai chi, or whatever practice you do. Notice your breath as you inhale and exhale during your workout.

Each of these ordinary activities has a positive effect on our physical and mental well-being, and each can make a difference. There is no reason to sit around and wait for something special. Face each task and each day with appreciation. When you do, you'll begin to notice the special in the ordinary.

32.

Sun-Faced Buddha, Moon-Faced Buddha

VALUING YOUR TIME

When Master Mazu fell ill, a monk came to ask
how he was feeling.
"Sun-faced buddha, moon-faced buddha," he replied.

MY BET IS that the monk had no idea what the hell he was talking about. Few people ever did. He was a rock star in the Zen world.

Old Mazu was well versed in the sutras, one of which mentions a sun-faced buddha who lives for 1,800 years and a moon-faced buddha who lives for a single day and night. For an awakened Zen master, there is no time; there is only the eternal now. A single day and night is no different in meaning or value than 1,800 years.

Master Mazu used the exchange to teach the monk that from an awakened perspective, being healthy or sick, feeling good or bad, living for a long time or for a short while are all relative states that arise and fall away.

They are all of the same temporary, fleeting nature. The master was not interested in how much time he had left. His focus was on being present, awake, and aware, which enabled him to face whatever was to come his way.

Have you ever thought about the expression "killing time"? Wasting time is one thing, but killing it? Wow, what an expression! Time is one of our most precious resources—as long as we think in terms of time, that is! Zen is about using our time for something meaningful rather than "killing" it.

When cancer comes calling, the value of even the smallest moment of time is magnified, and our appreciation of life quickly transcends its usual limited scope. When our view of life grows more expansive and more meaningful than simply how we feel on a given day, we naturally begin to make the most of the time that we have here, whether it is a single day and night, or 1,800 years. Mazu would certainly endorse this approach.

It is extraordinarily beneficial, and even necessary, to carve out some time, at least once a week, if not daily, when you can focus on taking care of just you and your needs. If you didn't already do this before cancer, you have all the more reason to do it now. The following exercise is meant to help you develop an appreciation of the time you have, and the motivation to use it well.

- Take a moment to reflect on the value of taking regular quality time to care for yourself.

- Decide when, during the day or week, you can set aside half an hour or an hour just for yourself and your rejuvenation. An easy way to create "extra time" is to reclaim some of the time we spend watching television or surfing the Internet.

- Set aside a precise chunk of time each day or week that you will spend on "personal rejuvenation time." Write it down in your calendar or on a piece of paper as a reminder. Think of it as an act of self-care and self-respect.

- Choose a specific exercise from this book (or another rejuvenating exercise that appeals to you) to practice during the time you have set aside.

- You could also use this precious time to read something spiritually uplifting, to take a long, relaxing bubble bath, to meditate, to exercise, to create some art, to take a walk somewhere beautiful, or to do any other activity that settles your mind and supports rejuvenation.

- Write down a list of activities you would like to do, and preserve your daily or weekly practice, as an act of self-love and self-respect.

You can always add to the list or change the time, but honor yourself by keeping that extra time for the things that bring you the most joy, healing, and peace of mind. When we juggle work, family, and cancer treatments, even a short amount of time devoted solely to caring for ourselves can feel like a lifetime. That little pocket of set-aside time is where we transform ourselves from a moon-faced buddha into a sun-faced buddha.

33.
A Drifting Fishing Line

MEDITATING WITH WATER IN NATURE

*"The Boat Monk" was a monk who ferried folks across
the Wu River in old Shanghai. He freely admitted that
he would have made a lousy abbot, because he enjoyed
the freedom of the great outdoors too much to give
it up. Over the years he became very well known
for words of wisdom such as, "If you only row in the
clear waves, it's hard to find the golden fish," and,
"Fish seen in clear water won't take the hook!"*

THE BOAT MONK taught us to let our minds drift, like a
fishing line, bobbing and floating, being and observing.
It is the nature of water to cool, to moisten, to ground,
and in the absence of big waves, to calm. We can even
use cooling, calming water as the basis for an awareness
exercise.

This exercise can be practiced near a body of water. In
the absence of a river, a lake, or another body of water,
this is one exercise that could take great advantage of a
rainy day. This is a wonderful mindfulness practice that

uses nature to soothe our senses, calm our minds, and relax our bodies. It also gives us something productive to do when it is raining outside and going out feels like too much of a chore—we can make productive use of the rain instead.

- Find a dry area near the water, or on a dry porch or near an open window looking out into the rain.
- Settle into a comfortable sitting position and connect to your breath.
- Allow your whole body to relax as you feel your breath enter and fill your belly and as you exhale through your nose.
- As you continue to breathe, notice how your body moves with each inhale and exhale.
- As you begin to relax, shift your gaze to the water.
- While continuing to breathe, relaxing, notice the ripples, reflections, sounds, colors, and even smells of the water.
- Allow your awareness to become enveloped by the sensory qualities of the water, yet remain mindful of your breath.
- Allow your sense of self to disappear and your mind to drift and connect with the liquid, flowing quality of the water.
- Rest in this calming meditation as long as you like.

A new monk said, "Master, please show me the gate where I can enter into awakening."

Master Xuansha said, "Hear the sound of the water in Yan Creek?"

The monk said he did.

"That's the place of your entry," the master replied.

34.

Boil Some Tea

DEVELOPING A MINDFULNESS RITUAL

A monk asked Master Cuiyan,
  "What is the most profound teaching you offer?"
The master called to his attendant,
  "Come and boil some tea!"

THE TEA CEREMONY is one of the traditionally revered arts of China and Japan. It is seen as an exercise in Zen mindfulness and even as a potential means to enlightenment. Chinese and Japanese tea rituals are designed precisely to allow the tea lover to appreciate all of the sensory aspects of tea—the color, aroma, taste—and the many sensations of drinking the tea itself. To truly appreciate tea, you must slow down and take a conscious break from your busy life. This can be your daily cup of mindfulness.

We don't have to wear a special kimono to create our own personal tea ceremony. Yes, a private pagoda overlooking a koi pond is a nice touch—but fortunately not required. A personal tea ceremony can be a way of stepping outside of our busy lives, to create a mindful pause between what we were just doing and what we will be doing later. The tea ritual provides a moment of escape from what is going on around us. Master Jiashan was the first Zen master to connect the Way of Tea with Zen. He is known for the four-character phrase: "Zen, tea, one taste!"

Making a cup of tea provides a great opportunity to practice meditative mindfulness. If we calm our minds, and focus simply on placing the tea leaves or tea bag into the cup or pot, pouring the hot water over the tea, watching tea leaves unfurl as they soak, smelling the aroma of fresh tea, feeling the warm cup in our hands, and savoring the taste of the tea, our nervous systems will also naturally be able to relax and recharge.

While it doesn't really matter whether we use fine china or a cracked old mug, a teapot, mug, and strainer that we find aesthetically pleasing can contribute quite a bit to our experience of the tea ceremony. The more attractive and satisfying we find our tea accouterments, the more likely we are to enjoy using them or to want to make performance of our tea ceremony a part of our daily routine. If you find tea ceremony to be an effective mindfulness practice for you, I recommend acquiring a cup and teapot that really makes it your own. Think of it as an investment in your daily mental and physical care.

If you prefer to use tea bags, find a mug or teacup that speaks to you. If you prefer to steep loose-leaf tea, look for a three-piece set that includes a mug, a filter, and a lid.

Choose a cup with colors that you find pleasing and relaxing, and with a shape that feels good and fits your hands.

It only takes a few moments of mindfulness to create your own daily tea ceremony:

- First, boil the water. Get your tea mug and tea while you wait for the water to boil. When the water is just about to boil, take it off the heat. (Never use boiling water for green tea—it is too hot and can scorch the leaves, which diminishes the flavors in the tea.)
- If you have never brewed loose tea before, I highly recommend that you try. Loose tea is always of higher quality than that found in tea bags, and the taste is far better and more complex. Good tea is like good wine. With good tea, you can experience many levels of tea flavors, such as fruity, floral, creamy, and sweet.
- If you are using loose tea, place the tea leaves in a filter or paper tea sleeve/sack.
- Before you pour the water over your tea bag or leaves, take a moment to close your eyes and just breathe. Take a few good, deep breaths and set aside any concerns, worries, or thoughts about plans. Bring yourself into the present moment. The present moment is always the only time you can experience the smells and tastes of your tea. If your mind is elsewhere, you will miss out on the full experience of "Zen, tea, one taste."

- Pour the water over your tea. Tea bags should only be left in for about a minute (follow the instructions on the box). Loose tea can brew up to a few minutes.
- Observe the water as it is infused by the color of the tea. Continue to breathe in a relaxed manner, with your head as free from chatter as you can throughout this meaningful little ceremony.
- When the color looks right, take the tea bag out of the mug and smell the aromas of the tea. Try to see if you can find any words to describe what you smell.
- Mindfully sip the tea. Maintain your awareness on each sip of tea.
- Take your time and never rush to finish. With each sip, feel the warm tea in your mouth and follow the sensations after you swallow. Note how the taste may be different from the aroma, or even different from the day before. Savor each moment as you savor your tea.

Always find a comfortable, relaxing place to enjoy your tea. Create an oasis of calm while paying attention to all of your senses. Try to maintain a state of mindful awareness sip after sip, day after day.

35.

Crawling Turtles

OPENING TO WHAT COMES

A monk named Guo once complained,
"When I went to the master with my question, I
expected an answer like a galloping horse,
but I got a crawling turtle instead."

LET'S THINK ABOUT what it means to be "a running horse" or "a crawling turtle." A horse may get someplace faster, but the turtle has the time to figure out whether it is indeed approaching the place it wants to be. There are pros and cons to each; whether one is "better" than the other is missing the point.

Only a valuating mind, an expectant mind, a judging mind favors the horse over the turtle, or the turtle over the horse. Sometimes life gives us a galloping horse and sometimes it gives us a crawling turtle. Most of the time we do not get to choose which. We might often be lost too deeply in our own drama to be able to see life's horses and turtles objectively.

When we expect a horse and get a turtle—as when,

for example, a scan returns with mediocre results when we expected fantastic improvement—expectations will ultimately have to be adjusted to the reality that confronts us. This need not be such a bad thing. How can we learn to bend like a reed in the wind if there is no wind?

Monk Guo went to his teacher with his "preferential mind." He approached his teacher with particular expectations, which, being a great Zen master, his teacher did not fulfill. The monk was let down, but he had an opportunity to let go of expectations and open to the unexpected. There is such great freedom in letting go of things having to be your way.

This "preferential mind" is our everyday mind on autopilot. It evaluates and judges everything that happens to us in life. It takes no effort to do this; we simply do it by habit. When we get wrapped up in our own judgmentalism, we become resistant to the many opportunities that life presents us when things aren't what we want them to be. Initially, Monk Guo did not feel that he got what he came for when he went to his master, but we can see that he got what he needed. He was forced to reconsider his view, to open to what the present presents, and then return to his master once he understood how to let go of preferential mind.

It is inevitable that our expectations will occasionally be out of sync with reality. We may want to be finished with a treatment protocol sooner than is possible, or we may want to escape to a desert island somewhere.

Aversions and desires like these are unlikely to affect the outcomes (unless you own a desert island), but they are quite likely to drive you crazy if you fixate on them—especially when something can't be changed. The practice of Zen encourages us to let go and accept that sometimes we must do what we must do, and then get on with it.

Let go of trying to turn turtles into horses. Greet and welcome each experience exactly as it is. Let go and experience the freedom that results from accepting what you cannot change, whatever it may be.

36.
Dig Inside

PRACTICING INTERNAL FOCUS

Master Dazu said, "It's better to dig one foot down into yourself than to spread Dharma ten feet wide outside."

DHARMA IS THE Sanskrit word for the teachings of the Buddha. Reading about and discussing Dharma are great ways to supplement our practice from the outside, but without attending to our inner garden we don't really have a practice. Master Dazu believed that our time was better spent cultivating the ability to experience our true inner nature, rather than spending that time spreading the teachings, without the actual experience of them. In other words, it is more meaningful and useful to be yourself than to be a parrot.

Our inner garden, or inner landscape, needs tending if we are to experience who we truly are and develop the ability to be able to think and act from this place. If you've been feeling edgy, easily distracted from what matters, or if things or people have been getting on your nerves more than usual, it is time to turn your focus inward and do a little digging.

Sometimes our feelings are covering up other feelings that we are trying to avoid! It may be easier for some of us to get angry than to admit that we feel sad or let down. It may be easier for some of us to cry than confront someone who did us wrong. We all have places in our lives that we unconsciously avoid giving too much awareness to. These places remain in the shadows, in the dark unknown. The more in touch we are with who we truly are—joyful, free, selfless, and pure—the more those shadows recede.

It is important to do some internal weeding from time to time. We need to regularly examine ourselves to be aware of what hidden internal factors may be contributing to our moods and reactions to life's challenges. For example, if something has been "triggering" you, causing you to become reactive, emotional, or irrational, that may be a sign that your inner shadows require some attention. Unless and until you are willing to take a good look at what's beneath your reactivity, you will continue to lose your cool without knowing why.

Triggers can come in many forms. Sometimes even an innocent and well meaning "How are you holding up?" might set us off. I know at times I've felt like taking people who ask me that by the shoulders and yelling, "How the hell do you think I'm holding up?!" Snapping at small stuff like that may happen because we're tired of being asked the same question over and over, or because we're tired, or because we're scared of how we're actually doing. The truth is that when we avoid how we feel about things, and push our feelings deep into the shadows of our mind, we might explode at anything that reminds us of what we hope to not face.

But once you unpack what is beneath your reactivity, you begin to feel better almost immediately. It only takes a moment to step back from a situation, look honestly at your reactivity, and then question yourself about why this reaction arose. With continued practice, we can get in front of our triggers and defuse them before we snap at our friends, family, or doctors.

- As soon as you feel an emotional response being triggered, stop right where you are.
- Don't speak or move.
- Breathe deeply and evenly, letting go of tension you might be holding in your body.
- Turn your awareness away from the trigger, inward, toward your reacting mind.
- Observe your inner landscape and listen to the message behind or beneath your reaction: what is it really about?
- Try to assume a dispassionate perspective toward your feelings and reactions. Remember that feelings come and go, like clouds in the sky, if we let them.
- Breathe a bit and practice these reflections before taking any external action, such as speaking. When

you can, take as much time as you need to sit with your hidden fears or anger to unpack them and bring them out of the shadows.

I find that even a few seconds of breathing and introspection are enough to change how I feel about the situation before I react to it out of hand. This type of internal focus is easier to practice with lesser triggers first. In lieu of practicing in the moment, you may find it helpful to practice when nothing is immediately bothering you. In such cases, you may simply think about or recall a situation in which you lost your cool and went off on someone. The more you practice this, the greater your reserve of patience will be when you encounter the stuff that really drives you bonkers.

When you turn your awareness within, you give yourself the time and space to change your mind, which will immediately change your mood. At the very least, you can shed a little light on why you have been moody about something. Master Dazu would say that we only have something meaningful to discuss after we've practiced being quiet and checking in with ourselves.

Digging inside is better than flinging dirt around outside!

37.

Like an Arrow

WALKING MEDITATION OUTDOORS

It is said that a Zen master can be so present
and in tune with her environment that if
someone were to shoot an arrow at her,
she could catch it in her teeth.

I'LL TAKE their word for it. ·

While it takes a bit of practice to be able to embody this level of presence and engagement with our environment, we can cultivate an enhanced sense of attunement right where we are. Walking is a normal part of almost every day, but chances are we usually do it in a rushed or distracted way. "I've got to get to the doctor! I've got to meet the kids at school!" But walking can also be used as an opportunity to slow down, to be present, and to observe the moment.

Once cancer comes along, we realize how fortunate we are when we have it in us to take ourselves for a stroll outside, even if it is only around the block. Walking, as a simple exercise for developing awareness of our environment and acknowledging what is, is a fabulous place to begin mindfulness practice. The only time you can appreciate what you have is right now, after all.

Normally, time zips past, like an arrow loosed from a bow—day breaks and fades into darkness, weeks and months fall away, seasons melt one into the other without cease. It can seem as if life is flying by. One thing on which physicists and Zen Buddhists agree is that there is no such thing as linear time. All we have to work with is the never-ending NOW. Unfortunately this is not naturally evident to us. Instead, we spend most of our moments thinking about or planning for other moments. Much of our suffering comes from our worries and preoccupations with a hypothetical future that exists only in our minds. Wise masters warn us that since this very moment is what we have at our disposal, we must pay attention right now!

When the weather is fine and you've got the energy, take advantage of that moment to get your arse out into nature. Such are perfect times to practice paying attention. Plus, you know that the exercise will do you some good! Most of us feel noticeably different in nature. We are able to relax a bit more, and our senses of sight, sound, touch, and smell are all enjoyably stimulated by it. Being out in nature helps us to feel more connected to everything around us—to feel "a part of" our surroundings. It also gets us out of our heads and our habitual thinking, which helps open us up to a wider perspective.

- Go somewhere beautiful and fit for taking a stroll—you know the place.
- Leave judgment behind when you leave for your walk; leave discriminating thoughts behind.
- Walk with no agenda.
- No cell phone; no iPod.
- Be a pure witness, taking everything in without labels.
- Allow your focus to settle on what surrounds you, rather than on whatever thoughts may arise.
- Note the colors around you. Do the trees have leaves? Are the flowers in bloom? Or if you are in a city, what types of people or stores are you walking past?
- Take in the smells. Stop and smell the roses, literally. If there are no roses, find a flower to smell on your walk today. Jasmine is abundant in San Francisco, and its aroma can fill the air for an entire block.
- Listen to the sounds around you. Are there any birds singing? Wind rustling through the trees? Children playing?
- At some point, bring your awareness to your feet. What does the ground feel like underfoot? Change textures on occasion by walking on grass, on a sandy beach, or on a dirt hiking trail.
- With each step, try to keep your awareness on what you are doing, feeling, smelling, listening, and seeing right NOW.

If walking is too much, try this exercise sitting on a bench in a natural setting. You can still use all of your senses and become more attuned to your environment.

Something special, even magical, happens when we let go of our thoughts and steep ourselves in our environment. We become a part of the walk, rather than the agent at its center. If you make walks like this a regular habit, the passing of the seasons will slow, so that you can fully admire their every unique moment. Time will no longer fly by like an arrow.

III.
Harnessing Your Mind

38.

Worthy!

USING POSITIVE MANTRAS

Once, when asked to confirm another's Zen
mastery, Master Daowu shouted, "Worthy! Worthy!"

THIS IS AN EXAMPLE of a beautifully positive mantra bestowed by a master on a student. A mantra is a sacred verbal formula repeated to invoke a certain state of awareness and to aid in meditative concentration. Many of us habitually and unconsciously repeat to ourselves what I call "negative mantras." We tell ourselves "I'm not good enough," or "I'll never be able to do that." There is no limit to the creativity we show in coming up with negative mantras!

Unfortunately, we tend to believe our thoughts, regardless of how capricious they may be. As a result, the more we repeat negative mantras to ourselves, the more likely we are to see ourselves according to their negative content. This is why positive mantras are so helpful. We can use positive mantras to replace unconscious pessimistic habits with conscious healthy thought patterns.

It is even more important that positive mantras well up from inside ourselves. We must use our inner Zen master to remind ourselves that we are indeed worthy. Mantras that emerge from the depths of our own minds are truly powerful.

It can be easy to succumb to pessimistic thinking when the odds are not in our favor, or when things don't seem to be going as smoothly as we'd hoped. It is easy, but not particularly beneficial. I find positive mantras particularly helpful during treatments, such as receiving an infusion or getting acupuncture. During a treatment, I might repeat the thought, "My body is healthy, strong, and radiant," or "This treatment is healing every cell." After qigong, I will take a few moments and repeat the thought, "With each breath I am healing and whole."

- The trick to finding an effective mantra is to allow it to emerge naturally from a place of deep positive thought and self-support.
- Use the mantra to replace and counteract negative or pessimistic ruminations.
- Using the mantra is an act of kindness: give yourself a positive word or short sentence to lift yourself up.
- Find a mantra that you can recite when doubt creeps in, or even better, a mantra that helps to keep doubt out. Make sure the mantra is a positive affirmation that will help keep your spirits up.

- Try to use active words to make the mantra more powerful: Instead of "I can do this," try "I am doing this!"

  Here are some of the mantras I have used:
  "I am worthy."
  "I am enough."
  "Thank you for my complete and durable healing."
  "My energy is strong and my mind is peaceful."
  "I am making it through with flying colors."
  "Thank you for the many parts of me that are strong, vibrant, and healthy."

Repeat the mantra silently in your head or out loud to yourself. Let your mind embody the sentiment of the mantra. Make the repetition of the mantra a moment to treat yourself with positive regard. The more you repeat the mantra, the deeper its meaning will take root in your psyche. Only you have the power to manifest your mantra.

You are most definitely worthy!

39.

A Fallen Flower
Doesn't Return to the Branch

BEING HERE NOW

A fallen flower
returning to the branch?
Ah, a butterfly!
—MORITAKE

ONCE A FLOWER falls, it doesn't try to figure out how to get back to its branch. It doesn't wonder whether it should have fallen in a different spot or beat itself up over how it could have fallen better. Flowers, unlike us, are blessedly free from insecurity and self-doubt.

It is easy to second-guess the decisions we make concerning our cancer: Should I have chosen option A or option B? Was that other doctor a better fit? Should I have kept working? Should I have spent $2,000 on that magical butterfly tongue elixir to help my hair grow back quicker?

When it comes to decision-making regarding cancer, it is rare that our vision is 20/20, even in hindsight. There are myriad factors to consider for each decision; some known, some still unknown, and some that we may never be able to know. As mere mortals, all we can do is make the best decision given the information we have at the time. Once we've left our branch it is out of our hands. We must let go and see where the wind takes us.

The Zen-like poet Robert Burns wrote, "The best laid plans o'mice and men often go awry." Mice and men; oncologists and their patients. Life will unfold as it does, despite our most intricate and careful planning. This thought may be frightening, but it allows for happy accidents and "learning opportunities."

- When things fail to go as hoped or according to plan, "should'ves" and "could'ves" aren't going to change it.
- Drop them. Let them go. They're not real. They are only fantasies.
- We needn't cling to what could've been.
- All we have is this moment, right now. So, "What now?"

We cannot return a fallen blossom to its branch. We cannot go back in time. What we can do is open our eyes, take a deep breath or two, and figure out where we go from here.

What NOW?

40.

Everyday Mind Is the Way!

WRITING LITTLE POEMS

Master Linji (Rinzai) saw the same potential
  in all everyday activities:
"Just act ordinary, without trying to do anything
  in particular. Move your bowels, urinate, get dressed,
  eat your rice, and if you get tired, lie down."

MANY ZEN MASTERS are not only able to find the special in what is ordinary, they are able to turn the ordinary into a spiritual path. What can we do to make the ordinary extraordinary? We can simply embrace the wonder of our "everyday mind." Master Linji encourages us to take a poetic approach to daily life.

Writing haiku poetry is a great, creative way to practice everyday mind. We don't need to be artsy-fartsy, and the difficult, rhyming language of Shakespeare is greatly discouraged in haiku. The haiku poet observes what is special about commonplace objects and settings—things we are typically too busy and inattentive to have even noticed. The poet attempts to capture the uniqueness of the everyday in just three lines: one of five syllables, then one of seven, and lastly another of five. You don't have to stick to the 5-7-5 syllable rule, though. Instead, use them as guidelines to keep your poems short and to the point.

Rather than relying on flowery or saccharine descriptions, the poet imbues the lines with beauty and emotion in the simple way that she presents the image. The hidden benefit of writing haiku is that for the few poetic moments spent shaping the lines to reflect the simplicity of nature, our minds grow focused on the natural world around us, and the recurring inner script of hope, fear, and doubt is put on hold.

While you don't need to leave your house to write haiku, I find a change of scenery to be the perfect spark for my creative, poetic mind. Haiku are usually about nature, so find a place outdoors—somewhere visually stimulating, for example. Haiku poems describe something ordinary, from our everyday lives, and present it in such a way as to create a feeling of emotion, such as sorrow, yearning, or happiness, in the reader.

- First find a good place to sit that affords you a dynamic vantage point on the scene. If you can't get outside, find a comfortable place inside that gives you a view outside or of the interior setting of your house that might include family members, housemates, or pets.
- Take a few deep and even breaths, and allow your

mind to settle into a state of open concentration—relaxed but present and alert to everything around you.

- Allow yourself to simply observe the scene.
- When something in the scene moves you, causing a feeling to arise in you, take that as your subject. Perhaps you encounter a bird you've never seen before, or a flower catches a bit of sunlight and speaks to you. Or perhaps the sound of the wind or a bird's song sparks a memory.
- Now, rather than describing how you feel, use words to paint a clear picture of what you've observed. Rather than describing the feeling that the cries of baby birds to their mama calls up in you, focus on describing the cries of the birds such that the image speaks for itself.

The goal in writing haiku is to conjure the scene in the mind's eye of the reader such that the reader experiences the same feeling you did when observing it.

One of the first haiku poems I had published was:

cold stone bench—
a fly & i
rubbing our hands
(from *Modern Haiku*, 1996)

This poem, like all of my poems, does not conform to the 5-7-5 syllable rule, and yours needn't either. There is no "right way" to capture a moment with poetry. Play, experiment, be open to rewriting and revisiting your poems. Enjoy yourself and appreciate the time spent paying attention to your surroundings.

Of course you need not wait until you are feeling poetic to notice that the ordinary is indeed extraordinary. Routine acts practiced with mindfulness can be extraordinary. Whether our daily tasks are nothing special or something extraordinary simply depends on our everyday mind. Everyday mind is the Way!

41.

Go Wash Your Bowl!

TAKING ACTION TO CHANGE YOUR MOOD

A monk asked old Master Zhao to teach him.
Old Zhao replied, "Go wash your bowl!"

EVEN THE SIMPLEST things, like doing the dishes, can be a means of waking up to the truth of who we are. It all comes down to our mindset.

When we feel peaceful, washing a bowl is a pleasant task (or at least it is quick and easy). On the other hand, when we are in a funk, washing a bowl can feel like too much work.

We have all had our share of days when it is tough to muster a positive attitude. When we have a bunch of these days in a row, we may have fallen into a funk. The blues can come without warning.

What's the best thing to do when we have the blues or the blahs? The Zen answer is as simple as washing a bowl: Anything.

Anything?

Anything!

Get up; put one foot in front of the other; do one small thing that needs doing. Water the plants. Mail a letter. If you don't have enough energy to get out of bed, return a friend's phone call, open a book, practice deep breathing. Anything!

It is easier to keep a ball rolling once you get it rolling. When we have the blues, it is hard enough to do something, much less to assume the "correct" or "mindful" attitude when doing it. But even the smallest action can help break us out of a funk. So begin with the first part— the doing something. Take that first step to get the ball rolling again. Once we are on our way, it is a little easier to keep going.

What small step can you take to shake off a funk?

Go wash your bowl!

42.
When to Pick Up Your Nose

LAUGHTER IS THE BEST MEDICINE

A monk asked Master Yunmen,
   "What is the purity of all-encompassing wisdom like?"
Yunmen spat at him.
The monk said, "How about some
   teaching method of the old masters?"
Yunmen replied, "Come here! Cut off your feet,
   replace your skull, and take away the spoon
   and chopsticks from your bowl. Now pick up your nose!
The monk said, "Where would one find
   such teaching methods?"
Yunmen yelled, "You windbag!"
   And struck the monk with his staff.

ONE OF THE MOST refreshing things about Zen is that it welcomes and appreciates humor. In Zen we use humor as a teaching tool. Laughter helps us not take ourselves and our precious egos so seriously. Humor is also a way to express one's insight and understanding, or as in the above case, to poke fun at a questioner's lack of insight or understanding.

In the above passage, a monk wanted to get all of the answers to his big spiritual questions from Master Yunmen. A Zen master like Yunmen would find this ridiculous. Yunmen knew well that there is no way to simply teach truths that must be experienced for oneself. If the monk had been awake, had experienced a taste of his true self, he would have known that the answers to these questions are only found through one's own experience.

Yunmen would not cater to this beginner monk and instead responded to the monk's earnest but misplaced questions in spontaneous and humorous ways. His responses escalate in their absurdity, to reflect the absurdity of the monk's thought. This little story illustrates how humor can help when we are in over our heads, or when we need to stop taking ourselves so seriously.

My mother, who has also undergone cancer treatments, told me that sometimes when people at her oncologist's would say, "You look so good!" my mom would reply, "Yes, I guess cancer agrees with me!" I find myself, too, bringing out the absurdity of the mundane questions put to me in treatment like "Can I get you anything?" "Yes! A double cheeseburger, fries, and a shake please!" My attitude tends to get a laugh or a smile, which I happily share in. In case you haven't noticed, smiling is contagious! Having a good sense of humor comes in handy when you have cancer. Yes, we can laugh and smile when we have cancer, and we most certainly should, as often as possible.

Why laugh? Because studies show that laughter reduces your stress hormones and increases the response of immune cells. Laughter provides a workout for your body's core muscles, increases blood flow and oxygenates the blood, and acts as an analgesic to reduce pain. Laughter also improves alertness, creativity, and memory. Would you believe that it takes less than a second for the health benefits of laughter to start to kick in?* Seriously!

It is easy to find ways to laugh. Part of the trick is to remind yourself of this by keeping in touch with what made you laugh before cancer. I have a good friend, for example, with whom I can share a good laugh even at my own expense. We all have friends or family members who help us let our guard down and not take ourselves so seriously. Keeping in touch with the people, movies, books, or ideas that help us to laugh at life is an important part of helping ourselves get healthy.

---

*If you are interested in the details, see: M. P. Bennett and C. Lengacher. "Humor and Laughter May Influence Health: III. Laughter and Health Outcomes," *Evidence-Based Complementary and Alternative Medicine*, (March 2008): 37–40, doi: 10.1093/ecam/nem041; M. P. Bennett, J.M Zeller, L. Rosenberg, and J. McCann. "The Effect of Mirthful Laughter on Stress and Natural Killer Cell Activity," *Alternative Therapies in Health and Medicine* 9(2) (March–April 2003): 38–45; L. S. Berk, D. L. Felten, S. A. Tan, B. B. Bittman, and J. Westengard. "Modulation of Neuroimmune Parameters During the Eustress of Humor-Associated Mirthful Laughter," *Alternative Therapies in Health and Medicine* 7(2) (March 2001): 62–72, 74–76.

- Spend time with that friend who helps you laugh at the absurdity of life. With cancer comes a host of new friends with cancer that you meet along the way. Many times you'll find that exchanging stories of the absurd situations you find yourselves in is a source of much laughter.

- Embrace the "interesting" changes in appearance that you go through with humor: why not wear a fun hat to cover your bald head, or get a temporary henna tattoo when you go bald? It's okay to chuckle at the strangeness you see looking back at you in the mirror. When you look funny, you look funny! When I began to grow my hair back, it grew in curlier than it had ever been. It was so curly that I looked like I was wearing a steel wool pad on my head, or that I had the world's worst Jew-fro. This hairdo gave me months of laughter until it finally grew out and settled down.

- Listen to comedy routines, see a funny movie, or read a humorous book (David Sedaris did wonders for me).

- Find what makes you laugh, and make regular use of it.

Over the years it has become very easy to laugh at myself—I have had tons of opportunities to practice and hone this skill. If Zen masters find it perfectly appropriate to use humor when words can't take us where we want to be, then there's no good reason why we cancer patients shouldn't follow in their wise footsteps.

Ha!

43.

Contentment Is True Wealth

ACCESSING INTERNAL WEALTH

Ryokan famously said,
"Contentment is true wealth!"

A POET-MONK, Ryokan was an outdoorsy type, known for playing in the fields with local children while out begging and teaching. When he spoke the above line, he was likely quoting the Dao De Jing, which says that to know contentment is wealth.

Bills can sure pile up quickly when you have cancer. This is especially so if we are no longer working, or if we pursue extra help with our healing outside of the oncologist. Meditation and qigong classes cost money, herbs and supplements cost money, and the list goes on. Our worries about the cost of surviving can seem overwhelming, whether or not we have cancer.

But let's not groan about money. Instead, let's take Ryokan's observation to heart. He reminds us that inner wealth is not dependent on our bank balance. In fact, these days we have more control over our inner wealth than we do over our outer wealth. And our inner wealth can be very useful when facing health challenges.

Inner wealth is revealed and expressed through gratitude for all that we have. There are so many things to be grateful for, many of which are so small and taken for granted that we may completely overlook them. Finding true wealth is about considering all that we have, rather than all that we want.

- At this very moment, look inside and find something that you are grateful for. It can be something big or just a little thing. You can think of a short list, or go with the one thing that sticks out the most in your mind. Maybe someone you know or love did something special for you. Maybe you are grateful for your own ability to do something for yourself or others. Let whatever gratefulness comes come.
- Focus your awareness on that feeling of gratitude.
- Let the positive feeling and sensation of gratitude fill your whole body; let it energize you, cell by cell.
- Allow your whole body and mind to feel enveloped by the feeling and sensation of gratitude. Take it one step further and feel grateful that you have this gratitude in your life!
- Spend a few moments to steep in the feeling of gratefulness that arises when you acknowledge what you have, rather than focusing on what you do not have.

- Breathe relaxedly and continue this reflection as long as you like.

Perhaps money isn't your greatest or most abundant asset these days. Fine. What is? You might be able to find practitioners willing to trade treatments or advice for a skill or asset (besides money) that you have to offer. In the meantime, you can always find true inner wealth when you turn your mind to the positive.

44.

Express Your Mind Without Your Tongue

CHANNELING EMOTIONAL ENERGY

Master Shouchu taught:
Language does not help matters.
Speech does not bring forth the truth.
Those who are burdened by language are lost.

ZEN VALUES ACTION over words and experience over eloquence. Words can point to the truth, but they are not the truth itself. Zen teaches us that emotions are temporary. Like clouds in the sky, we should simply notice them come and go rather than attach to them and get caught up in or perpetuate our own emotional dramas. This is much easier said than done.

For some of us, analyzing and talking through our emotions can be very therapeutic and cathartic. But for some of us, talking about our emotions is like stirring muddy water and brings no feeling of release. Even if you don't feel like talking about things, you can still help yourself feel better and move through emotional stuckness by moving your body in mindful ways.

Therapy wasn't really big in ancient China and feudal Japan. Zen masters learned how to channel their emotional energy and express themselves through teaching, art, music, tea, and martial arts, to name a few. None of these outlets depends on words, but all of them can help with pent-up feelings.

Tea ceremony is amazing to watch and learn, because every gesture and movement is brimming with mindfulness. From ballroom dancing and tai chi to knitting and cooking, moving your physical body while focusing your mind is a great way to channel emotional energy when words don't feel like the right avenue. I have friends who sew, who describe a feeling of peaceful tranquility that comes over them once they get into the flow of working on a particular piece.

My own outlet is the art of *shakuhachi*—the Japanese bamboo flute. The shakuhachi is difficult to play, and I don't necessarily always achieve a peaceful feeling or lose myself in the flow of practice. Nonetheless, because it is so difficult, playing it requires my full concentration and focus. I must be careful to get the tilt of the flute just right, to place my fingers in the proper positions for each note, and to blow in a way that creates the proper sound for each note, all while trying to read the music (in Japanese) correctly.

When I play the shakuhachi, there is no room left in my brain for thinking about anything other than exactly what I am doing at that very moment. This level of concentration naturally clears my mind. I couldn't even entertain stressful thoughts or get swallowed up in emotional drama if I wanted to! As an added bonus, the calm feeling and focused awareness I get from playing remains with me long after I put the flute down.

My mentor in Chinese medicine always told his anxious and worried patients to cultivate a hobby that required the use of their hands. A ridiculously large portion of your brain is dedicated to the movement of your first fingers and thumbs. Apparently it takes a lot of brainpower to be prehensile. Take advantage of this biological reality!

- Find a hobby that uses your hands to help focus your mind when you feel stuck and just don't feel like talking about it.
- Choose something you have a personal interest in, and which satisfies your creative or expressive urges.
- Set aside a regular piece of time to devote to your hobby. It is okay to let go and lose yourself in the flow of well-focused attention at work.

What does your wordless self-expression look like? Get your creative juices flowing in a way that involves your body and mind. When the mind and body move and flow freely, so do your emotions. No magic words required!

45.

Wisdom Shines through Darkness

WHO (NOT) TO SPEND TIME WITH

Wisdom banishes fear and ignorance,
just as light banishes darkness.

WE BECOME "enlightened" when we shine the light of wisdom on the areas of our consciousness that have remained hidden in the darkness of ignorance. Buddha said that to walk safely through the maze of human life, one needs the light of wisdom and the guidance of virtue.

What is wisdom? Wisdom is the knowledge gained from paying attention. Wisdom is taking the time to see through appearances. What's the difference between a voice of wisdom and reason and a voice of fear? Sometimes it can be difficult to tell, but it is helpful to learn how to recognize who's who.

As we journey through cancer, some people naturally become voices of reason. Others become voices of fear. I've noticed that cancer can be a great and powerful reminder to others that they too are mortal. It isn't easy for most people to think about life's biggest issues. As a result, well-intentioned friends and family members, worried for our health and well-being, may come to us with advice and warnings driven by their own fears. Most of these folks will not necessarily know what is reasonable in our situation, because they may not actually have (or understand) all of the details required to make an informed decision.

On the other hand, some friends and family members may be just what the doctor ordered. These folks often intuitively know what you need, whether it's the delivery of a meal, a shoulder to cry on, or just the right word at the right time. They too may be worried about you, but they don't let their worries overshadow their words and actions. Instead, they let their light shine in your presence to help banish your own darkness. The best people let virtue, rather than fear, guide their actions. These are the people who are eager, willing, and happy to be of whatever service is needed, no questions asked. I guarantee they're out there, and they may not be the ones you expected.

- If you are having a hard time determining if someone is a voice of wisdom or a voice of fear, shine some of your own wisdom on the situation.
- If you find yourself getting more freaked out or anxious after talking with someone, that is a red flag.
- A certain person may tend to ask only questions that have no answer, or discuss topics that provoke

greater worry about your health. If you have the same reaction time after time with a person like this, those are red flags piling up.

- Of course it is a difficult situation to be put in when we have to take our friend aside for the talk. No one wants to risk losing a friend, and this is doubly true when facing cancer!

- Center yourself and have a calm heart-to-heart conversation with such people to let them know how their way of approaching your situation makes you feel.

- If that doesn't work, and if such people simply cannot help themselves, you may need to ask that they give you your space for a while.

Know who your voices of wisdom are, and keep your light of wisdom shining brightly in their company. There is no reason to be overwhelmed by darkness, especially with the unwitting help of those around you. Shine the light of your wisdom, and cast away the darkness of fear.

46.

Thusness

ACCEPTING WHAT IS

My favorite Zen master once said,
"If you can't spank it, it isn't real."

LIFE DOLES OUT plenty of "what ifs," liberally sprinkled with "if onlys." Both reliably appear when we are in the mood to drive ourselves mad. "If only I had chosen treatment A instead of treatment B . . ." "What if I had listened to that other doctor?" These two are regular players.

It is time to let go of "what ifs" and "if onlys" that buzz around our heads like noisy bees. These types of distracting thoughts, unlike bees, are not actually even real. They have no basis in reality and have no bearing on what is happening at this moment. They are only noisy, harrying fantasies.

Thusness is a Buddhist word for the ability to stay in touch with reality. For something to demonstrate thusness it must exist right here, right now. Until there are time machines that allow us to see into the future or that can take us back into the past to try again, all we really have is what is in front of us right now. Is there something we can do at this point in time that can help or make a difference?

We can't change the past, but we can take steps right now that will positively affect our future. There is so much power in thusness—in being present and making decisions based on what we can do or change right now. Now is the only time in which we can make decisions or take action!

There is a quick, painless, and easy way to bring yourself back to "thusness" when you find yourself head-tripping over some possible future scenario, or replaying something from your past.

- Slow down, step away from whatever you were busy with.
- Breathe deeply and evenly, and let your focus settle only on the breath.
- Let your awareness settle into this moment, right now, following your breath in and out.
- When you have suitably settled into this very moment, simply ask yourself, "What can I do about this issue right NOW?"
- If there is something that can be done, collect yourself, and do it.
- If there is nothing that can be done, let it go with your out breaths.

The key to this practice is to accept what is, rather than freaking yourself out with what was or what could be. When you ask yourself this question, you immediately realize that you can't alter a thing from your past and you can't guarantee the future. If there is nothing that can be done now, you can give yourself permission to let it go and give it a rest.

After I began a chemo that is known to cause neuropathy (tingling and discomfort in the hands and feet), the neuropathy grew worse with each treatment. I kept imagining that in the not-too-distant future, I wouldn't be able to feel my patients' pulses (an essential part of the practice of Chinese medicine), pet my dogs without discomfort, walk on the beach, or even play flute. I kept picturing various future scenarios where I couldn't use my hands and where my feet were uncomfortable.

When I finally had enough of that, I began to study the condition, and found that L-Glutamine (an amino acid found in protein) can help with neuropathy. I bought the supplement and took it three times a day. After a month or two, the neuropathy improved so much that it disappeared from my hands completely. I can't even notice it in my feet unless I really try (I don't really try).

Of course there are times when the answer to a nagging question is, "No, I can't do a damn thing about it right now!" In those cases, take a few breaths and try to let it all go with your out breaths.

It isn't easy to keep your mind in the present, even

though there is usually plenty to occupy us in the present. But as with any practice, the more you test yourself with the question of "thusness," the easier it becomes to dispel these hallucinations and to focus on what is real and actually matters.

Now is always where you find your power. Now is always the time to act. Now is always the time of thusness!

47.
Stuck Like Ice

MOVING THE BODYMIND

Master Takuan likened a stuck mind to ice—
solid and frozen shut.

OUR MINDS should be like water, he taught, flowing
freely and easily with life's tides. The mind sometimes
behaves like a gerbil on a wheel, or like a dog with a
bone. Something gets in there and we can't stop it from
repeating over and over, like a broken record. We get
stuck thinking in a loop about heavy stuff, or about what
might happen next. Sometimes we get fixated on little
details; sometimes on big ones. Of course, occasionally
we really do need to think about these things, but without the repeat button.

Although there are many ways to thaw our minds
when they are frozen like ice obsessing over an issue,
one of the best and healthiest methods is to do something physically active to break the cycle. Exercise gives
us something else to focus on for a while, and releases
stress and tension, and thereby worry. From a Buddhist

point of view, the body and the mind are deeply inter-connected; in fact they are one. When you move your body you move your mind.

Being active also gives us a chance to get out with a friend. If you can, find a partner to join you in your chosen activity. Interaction with another also helps to keep us from fixating on the thoughts in our heads. I like to get outside when I need to thaw my frozen mind and clear my head. Taking hikes with my dogs near the beach usually does the trick. Sometimes I go alone so that I can keep a more internal focus, but sometimes I enjoy a little good conversation on these walks. Walking helps bring me into the present moment.

- Change your scenery, change your mind!
- Make a habit of getting out if you can.
- If you don't have the energy to go out, or the weather is not ideal, a little qigong may help get things unstuck (see the section on Self-Healing Qigong Exercises, on page 247 below). Tai chi and yoga also work well here.
- If something like qigong, tai chi, or yoga is too unusual for you, a good number of gentle stretching or exercise clips can be found on the Internet. Find one and try it out.
- If you have a friend who is game, schedule your outing or exercise together.

If you are having trouble moving your mind's energy, then it is a good bet that you need to move your body's energy. When you move your body's energy, you also move your mind's energy. Think of it as rebooting your nervous system. A regular habit of exercise is an excellent means of self-maintenance. Working with a partner is quite helpful, as we tend to find it harder to break an appointment with others than we do with ourselves. Make appointments with others to help you stay on track.

Call someone and make a date to do something active together. Or just get moving. Break through the ice!

48.
Baby Snake or Dragon?

EMBRACING STRENGTH AND VULNERABILITY

After observing his students, Master Nanquan
used to say that it was easy to tell the difference
between the dragons and the baby snakes:
Dragon students were powerful and unwavering,
and baby snake students were not.

THE TRUTH IS that we can be both dragons and baby snakes at various times and in various contexts. We are yang—powerful majestic dragons—and we are yin—vulnerable baby snakes. We cannot have yang without yin, or yin without yang. That would be like having only the front of a coin. Yin and yang are inseparable parts of the whole.

Junpo Roshi, a fellow cancer survivor, always says, "Your vulnerability is your greatest strength." When I was getting chemo, I found myself to be vulnerable, soft, and exposed. I became a baby snake. I didn't have the energy or the will to put up a valiant front. Instead, I chose to use what energy I had to get well, and as my strength came back, my inner dragon again returned.

Can you recognize both sides of yourself—the exceptionally strong side as well as the open, tender side? Both are always there, contextually dependent and equally valuable. We need to recognize that sometimes, like a mighty dragon, we feel powerful and invulnerable, but sometimes our energy wanes, and we feel like a baby snake.

Who we truly are transcends all that we are going through. But it's nice to remember that the principles of yin and yang always apply: where there is strength there is softness, and where there is softness there is strength. One does not, and cannot, exist without the other. We always have both.

Sometimes strength and energy are at our beck and call. At other times, strength is found in the recognition that we are vulnerable and need to rely on others for help. Learn how to ask for the help you need. You will feel so good about yourself for having the strength to do so. Have you been able to embrace the strength in recognizing your vulnerability? It helps.

Are you a baby snake or a dragon?

Yes!

49.
Sometimes the Obstacle
Is the Path

ACKNOWLEDGING ANY BENEFITS

Master Shoushan once held up a bamboo comb
before the monks and said, "If you say it's a bamboo
comb then you are grasping (to the form).
If you don't call it a bamboo comb, you're turning
away (from reality). So what will you call it?"

WHEN YOU BEGIN Zen koan practice, each koan feels
like an obstacle with no easy way of getting around it.
It stops you right in your tracks and your normal ways
of processing and thinking cannot help you to solve the
meaning underneath the Zen riddle. You can't answer
the above koan, or koans like "show me your face before
your mother was born," with your rational mind or your
sparkling intellect.

While each koan feels like a blockade, once it is solved,
it is actually a point of entry onto the path of experiencing
your true nature. Sometimes we must approach our challenges and mysteries with a fresh eye, a new perspective,

in order to find the true meaning in them. Cancer first appears as an obstacle on our path, which it very well may be, but it can also become a path itself.

A path to what? Well, more like a path "of what." Healing is both a path and a destination: it is something we want to be traveling through and something we want to reach. We can benefit tremendously by paying attention to the obstacles that this path must travel through, rather than only to its ultimate destination.

The path of cancer is comprised of many twists and turns, and there are many obstacles we must overcome along the way. Whether we realize it or not, this path intrinsically involves learning. We gain new understanding and new perspective along the way. How we face the many setbacks and challenges forces us to learn about ourselves, those around us, and life in general.

I'm not going to give you some sanctimonious spiel about how your cancer is a blessing in disguise. That is for you and you alone to decide. But what I will say is that I have gained deeper wisdom from my experiences with it by paying close attention to the many steps along the path of healing. Obstacles become the path when we are able to find a deeper meaning in them. Almost every life lesson comes with a hidden gem to discover; sometimes the gem is easy to spot, sometimes not.

When I was first diagnosed with cancer, my friends, students, patients, and family showered me with so much love and support I could hardly believe it. My students held a benefit for me at the school where I teach, and they gave treatments to the public to raise funds for me while I wasn't working. My friends brought us food, sent cards, sent gifts, and offered us all the help we could ask for. My whole family was by my side with love and support and no other agenda but to be of help. I didn't realize, or perhaps appreciate, how much love I had around me and how much my presence was appreciated by those I've touched. This was the first lesson for me on this path: to truly appreciate all the love in my life, and to appreciate the love I've cultivated in this lifetime. Every single day since then, without exception, I have acknowledged and appreciated all of the wonderful people and love around me. I felt and still feel blessed to know this depth and breadth of love.

Cancer has also taught me to slow way down. I used to be more of a Type-A, get it done quickly and efficiently type of person. Even in Chinese medicine school, I'd regularly go from a court hearing straight to a class and then back to my law office to write a legal brief. There were times I'd even rush through my morning qigong practice.

That type of rushing around felt normal to me. When I began to feel crappy and low-energy from the cancer treatments, I realized that I couldn't and didn't actually want to continue living at that pace. My motto has become "the slow lane has the best views." Not only is my nervous system more calm and relaxed, but I am much more mindful of each thing I do. No more multitasking for me! I've found that slowing down naturally helps me be more present, which has deepened my meditation practice. I also enjoy each thing I do just a little bit more; be it eating, sipping tea, driving, or spending unstructured time with friends.

I am what you might call a "mad optimist," so I can easily rattle on about how cancer has changed me for the better. I was a happy person before the cancer, and I am still a happy person, but now I appreciate that happiness much more. I don't take happiness, or anything else, for granted anymore. This is another of cancer's lessons for me: all-encompassing gratitude for what is good and right in my life.

You may find that you hate this cancer, or you may come to embrace it. This is your path, your journey. Regardless of your view of it or how you got here, you are now on a path you likely didn't expect to find yourself on. Will you take it on mindfully or mindlessly?

You may not end up as the same person you were before cancer came along. Many of us grow from the experience. It is hard to face something like cancer without having one's perspective changed. I feel wiser from living with cancer—though I'd have rather just seen the movie. The path has been filled with many obstacles, and sometimes even with gifts. I've tried my best to pay attention to each step, lest the learning pass me by.

- Use this very moment to take a brief inventory of your life as it is right now.
- It is perfectly fine and acceptable to acknowledge the difficulties and challenges you've faced since your diagnosis.
- For this exercise however, find something positive that you've come to learn, experience, understands or appreciate since you've been walking the cancer path. My bet is that there is at least one positive shift in your life that has resulted from the challenge of cancer.

Here's your koan for today: If you call cancer an obstacle, it is like putting frost on top of snow. If you don't call cancer an obstacle, then you are trying to smell a flower by cutting off your nose. So what will you call it?

50.

A Lustrous Pearl in Your Hand

APPRECIATING THE BEAUTY AROUND YOU

Master Jiashan said that when a dragon appears in the water, the fish don't notice the pearl in the dragon's mouth.

THEY ARE FOCUSED on the dragon and miss the pearl, an object of beauty and value. If you are like me, you probably spend quite a bit of time either thinking about your cancer, talking about your cancer, or doing something to help get rid of your cancer. We all can be like those fish—the dragon of cancer overwhelms our minds, and we forget the pearl in its mouth.

At my ordination, where I was given the dharma name Daju, or "Great Pearl," my sister priest Reishin gave a short talk on my new name. In that talk she reminded the gathering that every pearl begins as an irritation. Could she have been calling me an irritant? Likely.

Even cancer too can be like a pearl. It may begin as an irritant (and even continue as such), but it can help you find the pearls in life by paying attention to what is beautiful in yourself and in each situation that arises.

If the world is your oyster, then the beauty in your life is like the lustrous pearl part of you.

- Take a moment to recollect something beautiful that you enjoyed in your life from before your diagnosis: a painting, music, friends, an event, or a beautiful place. Give yourself space to really delve into and experience the memory. Continue until a smile comes to your face.
- Now, take a moment to reflect on something beautiful in your world today. Begin by looking out a window, or if you are reading this outside, look up. Take in the vibrancy of your environment—trees, flowers, birds, people, the buildings, the sky, the low din of traffic or of rain?
- Think of a beautiful relationship you have with someone right now—maybe a friend, a lover, a sibling, or a parent. Think about how that person makes you feel, or something special you've done with that person. Each loved one is like a precious pearl.
- Spend a bit of time in this way, letting your attention drift from the dragon to recognize the many pearls in its teeth.

There is still much that is beautiful to recognize, even in the jaws of the dragon of cancer! A lot may have changed since your diagnosis, but true, essential beauty is beyond the reach of sickness. It is only our distraction in the face of the disease that obscures the precious treasure in our lives.

Zen Master Baiyun composed the following poem:

> I possess a lustrous pearl
> long locked away by dust and toil.
> Now the dust is gone and a light shines forth,
> illuminating myriad blossoms, mountains,
> and rivers.

51.

Laughing Now

LETTING YOUR EMOTIONS FLOW

Master Baizhang said, "My crying before
is the same as my laughing now."

EMOTIONS CAN BE tricky. Even though feelings are only one of the ways that we take in information, we place great value on them. From a Zen perspective, feelings are no different than colors or sounds: they provide us with information. What we do with the information that they give us is another, usually more dramatic, story.

Master Baizhang understood this when he talked about crying and laughing. With a little thought, we can understand what the master meant. Both crying and laughing are physical manifestations of feelings. They are fundamentally the same. They appear like changes in the weather; they come and they go. Both will pass so long as we don't grasp on to them.

Laughing and crying also offer us a means of releasing pent-up emotional energy and stress from the body. Joni Mitchell agreed with Baizhang when she wrote and sang, "laughing and crying, you know it's the same release." Both are like pressure valves. Most of us could use a good cry or a good laugh, depending on the context. When the going gets tough, emotional meltdowns are bound to happen.

To be clear, I don't mean that we should be constantly overwhelmed and unable to cope with our emotions. If we find that we have grown consistently overwhelmed, depressed, anxious, and prone to uncontrolled crying or anger, we should of course seek out and rely on a qualified professional to help us recover and regain our balance. However, if from time to time we feel overwhelmed and break down in tears or break into laughter, that is pretty darn normal in our situation. I have had some wild, uncontrollable laughing fits since my diagnosis, and I've also had some wonderfully cathartic cries. I felt better after both.

- Give yourself permission to cry or to laugh when you need to.
- If you are shy about public displays of emotion, wait until you are alone to let it flow.
- Rent a funny movie or hang out with a funny friend who you know will make you laugh.
- Don't suppress your emotions. Letting them come up and out often makes room for rest and calm.

Allow yourself to experience the wisdom of Baizhang's words! Tears can become laughter, and laughter tears. Same, same.

52.

Bushido: The Way of the Warrior

COPING WITH WHAT ARISES

There is something to be learned from a rainstorm.
When meeting with a sudden shower, you try not
to get wet and run quickly along the road. But doing
such things as passing under the eaves of houses,
you still get wet. When you are resolved from the
beginning, you will not be perplexed, though you will
still get the same soaking. This understanding
extends to everything.

—YAMAMOTO TSUNETOMO, *The Hagakure: The Book*
of the Samurai

MANY OF THE ancient Zen masters and monks came
from the Japanese samurai class. Bushido, the code of
the samurai warrior, teaches that one must take no action
when angry or stirred by passions. This makes very good
sense when one is carrying a sharp and deadly weapon. It
also makes sense when one needs to be sharp for making
decisions following a cancer diagnosis.

There is nothing Zen about pretending everything is

okay when it's not. The path to inner peace requires honesty and wide-open eyes. The only way out is through, as the inspirational saying goes. Face what needs facing! The above quote from *The Book of the Samurai* uses how we hope to avoid rain as an example of how we hope to avoid facing reality. The author points out that when it rains, even though we hope to avoid getting wet, we will still get wet. If we just acknowledge from the beginning that rain is wet, and that we will therefore likely get wet when it rains, then we will not get upset when it happens. Such practical advice from a warrior!

The way of the warrior encourages us to look at what is in front of us and deal with it in an appropriate and constructive way, rather than let it get on our nerves, frustrate, and set us off balance. In other words, freak out for as long as you need to. Once that's out of the way, collect yourself and pick up your sword. It may feel like a challenge to find the coolest spot in the fire, or the calm in the storm. But the calm is always there; it is we who come and go with respect to it.

It is invaluable to know what will help you find your center when you get anxious, fired up, or can't think clearly. It is a good idea to develop a personal repertoire of practices or interventions that you can turn to in times of stress and emotionality. It may help to make a list for this purpose. Here are a few solid practices that have helped me:

- Take a brisk walk or jog to reset your mental thermostat.
- Do a bit of slow, deep breathing to relax your nervous system and to help you reboot.
- Take a little alone time, a little solitude to cool down. Maybe there is a local park or scenic view you like to frequent for this purpose.
- Rely on that close friend who gets you and doesn't mind letting you vent with him.
- Take a hike through the woods or along the beach to clear your head and regain your focus.
- In a pinch, take a few minutes to perform a full body-scan, relaxing each part of your body from your head down to your feet.

If you aren't already aware of what presses your "chill" button, now is the time to find out. Learning how to manage emotional reactions when they flare up helps us to quickly regain our composure, so that we can face whatever arises.

Life will give you plenty of opportunities to practice this, and you'll notice that once you get in the habit of doing a quick mental or emotional "reboot," clarity and calm come much more quickly and easily. You are not a victim of your own life; you are a warrior. Sharpen your sword!

53.
The Essence

NARROWING YOUR FOCUS

A monk asked Master Mazu,
"What is the very essence of Zen?"
The master replied,
"What is the meaning of this moment?"

WE FIND this kind of dialogue all throughout Zen literature. A student asks the master a very broad, philosophical question, and the master, in response, guides the student back to what matters: this very moment. The essence of Zen—and of our lives—is this very moment.

Why this moment? Because now is the only time when we can change our minds or take action. Now is the only time we can even think about taking action. All of our power to act resides entirely in this very moment. We can't take action in moments that have already passed or before they have arrived.

We sometimes get so caught up in trying to grasp the big picture we lose track of what is right in front of our noses. When the big picture starts to become overwhelming, bring your awareness to what is happening right now—to what is right in front of you. Let go of hopes and fears about what may come or about what has already passed you by. Attend to this very moment. It is easier to get a handle on the few things that you face right now.

When I feel overwhelmed by the thought of another chemo treatment, I remember Master Mazu and remind myself that I am not actually having the treatment at that very moment. These days, instead of letting my thoughts—just my thoughts—make me tense or upset, I now simply change my thoughts!

Living with cancer certainly presents its challenges, both physical and emotional. When fear or anxiety hits, it is so helpful to have the wherewithal to bring your mind back to the present. Most often, whatever you are worrying about is not happening in the present moment. Reminding yourself of this serves as a helpful reality check. In reality, the present moment is often just not that bad.

- If you find yourself worrying about your next scan or treatment, shift your focus and thoughts to the moment before you.
- Recall that you are not currently undergoing that treatment, and that any dreaded experiences associated with it are not actually happening now.
- Take in the scenery and enjoy the pleasure of being

with whoever you are with, rather than getting stuck in your head.

If you can return your focus to the present moment, whatever you are doing will shift in tone from a tense rumination on potential unhappiness to a relaxing, healing time with friends or with yourself. Ask yourself, "What is the meaning of this moment?"

54.

Your Nose

STEPPING AWAY FROM YOUR ROUTINE

Master Zhimen said,
"Your eyes can't see your nose!"

It may sound as if Zhimen is pointing out the obvious, but why can't your eyes see your nose? Because they're too close to it, of course. It is difficult to be objective when you are too close to something, or have too much invested in it. It is hard to see things in a new way when you've long been in the same routine without a break.

Isn't now the perfect time for a change of scenery?

Distance can often give us new perspective, which we can bring back to our daily grind. Distance can also give us space to breathe and to think about things outside of their usual context. Sometimes you don't even know that you need breathing room until you finally give yourself some.

Are you able to get away, if not literally, at least metaphorically? You needn't cross the entire country, or even leave your hometown. A short jaunt out of town, a visit to a beautiful park or botanical garden, or even a special night with an old classic movie can shake up our routine and get us out of our habit for a bit.

When my stomach decided that it was time to take a week off of chemo, I took advantage of the week off by road tripping through Portland, Oregon, to the Mount Adams Zen Temple in Trout Lake, Washington. Rather than sitting at home with my stomach pain, I had a great time with friends at a magnificent temple located at the beautiful Trout Lake Abbey.

I figured that if I had to have stomach pain, why not suffer somewhere beautiful? I believe that the trip helped speed the healing of my stomach, and the lull of the road helped clear my mind. I returned feeling ready to jump back into chemo and refreshed by the time I spent in nature.

- Carefully assess your energy levels. What do you need to do to "see your nose" more clearly?
- A day trip or a weekend get-away can really shift your perspective.
- If those are too much, call a good friend to get together and ask her for some advice.
- Take it to the next level by meeting her at a café or someplace new that you have never been to. Get creative.
- If you have the energy, visit a museum and bring home a souvenir as a reminder of your trip.

- If you really aren't up for an outing, transport yourself by watching one of those great, Vista Vision Hollywood classics at home.
- The more such outings break you out of your routine, the better.
- When you return, take a look at your daily life with new eyes—anything need changing? You can then use your fresh perspective to help change it!

It may be the perfect time to take a short or long road trip to a place you either love or have never been but have wanted to visit. Or, if you can't drive or fly somewhere beautiful, find an old nostalgic movie to watch, pictures to look at, or music to listen to. Find that special something that takes you to a different place in time, one that makes you smile or just gets you out of your head for a while.

55.

Losing Your Eyebrows

DOUBLE-CHECKING YOUR HABITUAL THOUGHTS

In China, Buddhist priests warned their students
that if they talked badly about Zen and Buddhist
teachings, their eyebrows would fall out.

CAN YOU IMAGINE what would happen if your eyebrows fell out whenever you've said something negative about yourself? How often do we find ourselves immersed in self-doubt or negative thoughts? How often are we truly aware of how we talk to others and ourselves?

"Right speech" is one of the eight essential steps on the Buddhist path, and it includes both spoken and unspoken words. Right speech is a spiritual practice. It is an act of self-love and mindful attention to thoughts and words. We can't change our tune to a more positive one unless and until we become truly mindful of our thoughts and words.

The next time you catch yourself in a downward spiral of self-doubt, or as I like to call it, "stinkin' thinkin'," take the opportunity to practice a little right speech.

- When you find yourself getting down on yourself or getting down on someone else, either in conversation or in thought, try asking yourself the following questions about what you have to say:
  - Is it true?
  - Is it necessary?
  - Is it kind?
- If what you think or tell yourself about yourself is not true, necessary, or kind, drop it immediately, just like that. Dropping such behavior right away is the only way you can change the way you think and speak. Likewise, if you find yourself in a conversation where what you are saying is not true, necessary, or kind, change it immediately. Drop it like the bad habit it is.

It is most important that we remember to apply the discipline of right speech to the way we think and talk about ourselves, as well as to others. Even if our eyebrows don't fall out when we talk or think negatively about others and ourselves, observing right speech reminds us that our thoughts and words have power. We get to choose whether we increase our inner positivity, and positivity in our relationships, or to let ourselves slide into negativity.

We can choose to bring positivity to others, and ourselves, even if our eyebrows will fall out anyway from chemo.

56.
Heads and Tails

FOLLOWING THROUGH

A common Zen chastisement:
"You have a dragon's head and a snake's tail."

WHAT DOES THIS MEAN? Well, a dragon is a mythical, mystical, massive, scaly, water or sky creature with magical powers; a snake is a small, or sometimes not-so-small, slithering, earthbound reptile. The master means to chide her student for having a great start but a weak finish.

Following through with our actions and continuing to do the things we love is even more important when it comes to dealing with cancer. The journey through cancer can go on longer than expected. Many of us put our lives on hold when we have cancer, and from my own experience, I can tell you that is a huge waste of our precious time here. When you live as if each day matters, you live like a dragon, and you do your best with whatever you choose to spend your time doing.

Obviously, sometimes you may not feel physically strong enough or well enough to participate in certain activities that you used to enjoy. Or there are certain activities you should avoid when you have cancer. It is a sad fact that you can't even have sushi or raw oysters when you are undergoing chemo, for example. Still, there is plenty out there that you can engage in to regain your sense of self-esteem and personal power.

It is easy to become more of a snake when undergoing cancer treatment. You can start out strong, but then the tiredness sets in, or your digestive system breaks down. You must always honor your limitations and work within your comfort zone and abilities. Regardless of how you've been feeling, this tip is all about reconnecting with the part of you that is a dragon; that fierce active presence inside you. We all have both aspects within us. It is important not to neglect one for the other. Find it in yourself to stay strong and healthily active as the time passes! Be a dragon!

You will need all of the energy you can get to keep working while fighting cancer. This being the case, it is even more important to return to some hobby or practice that gave you pleasure before cancer came along.

- Think of something that you began with a sense of enjoyment and enthusiasm but then dropped before finishing. We all have these projects. It could be something creative, like an art project, sewing, or remodeling a room in your house.
- Cook a nice meal to share with friends; or better yet,

have some friends bring food over for a potluck at
your home.

- If your energy is very low, use your time to visualize
the things you'd like to try or do in the future. Think
of a trip you'd like to take, or a person you'd like to
see, or an activity you'd like to try. Just visualizing
these can help boost your mood and energy. Even
if you can't act like a dragon, you can always stay in
touch with your inner dragon.

Master Dagui said that dragons and snakes are very easy
to tell apart, and of course he was right. You know when
you feel like a dragon and you know when you are feeling
snake-like. When you feel like a snake, it is easy to find
the excuses necessary to quit and slither away into some
hole in the ground. Time to be the dragon you are.

Dragon or snake? Heads or tails? What's your choice
today?

IV.

Balancing and Nourishing
Your Body

57.
Drink Some Tea!

STAYING HYDRATED

A disciple asked Master Zhao Zhou, "What is Truth?"
"Drink some tea!" he replied.

OLD ZHAO encouraged his students to find awakened mind in activities as commonplace as drinking tea. While he wasn't really advocating drinking tea, he was on to something way before it became a hip trend.

It is very important to stay hydrated when you're undergoing cancer treatment (and even when you're not). Green and black teas are a great way to stay hydrated, and they carry health benefits that only tea can offer.

Green tea is a well-researched medicinal herb. It is high in something called EGCG (epigallocatechin gallate). EGCG is a powerful antioxidant believed to have anticancer properties. Tea also has L-Theanine, which has been shown to calm the nerves and to activate enzymes in the liver to help rid the body of toxins. Who doesn't want that?

Find an organic tea that you enjoy and drink it without

adding dairy or sugar. Tea in bags is fine when you are on the go, but the best tea is never put in bags. Instead, it is kept as whole leaves and is brewed with special brewing apparatus called an infuser, which resembles a ministrainer.

Great tea is worth the price. Don't be cheap! You can make many cups of tea from a small amount of loose leaves, which makes it an economical buy in the end. Find a tea shop that supplies loose tea in your area or search online. For Chinese teas, start with jasmine pearl, or Formosa oolongs. For Japanese teas, Genmaicha and Kukicha will get you on your way. Nicer tea shops usually carry great tea gear too.

Japanese green teas may be richer in EGCG than Chinese green teas, but buy what tastes best to you, because that's what you'll actually drink!

58.

Three Pounds of Flax

KEEPING THINGS MOVING

A monk asked Master Tozan, "What is Buddha?"
Tozan answered "Three pounds of flax."

CANCER DRUGS can sometimes cause constipation. Chemo and pain meds often do too, as can antinausea meds. But lack of fiber or insufficient water in your diet can also cause uncomfortable constipation. It is important while healing to have regular bowel movements so that your body can properly absorb nutrients and get rid of wastes and toxins. Maybe Tozan understood this, as he apparently held flax in high regard!

Freshly ground flax works wonders when added to oatmeal, grains, or shakes. It helps to supplement your fiber intake to keep things moving smoothly. Grind it fresh so you don't lose nutrients such as healthy omega-3 fatty acids.

If you don't have an extra coffee grinder on hand to use for grinding fresh flax, substitute chia seeds, using them as you would flax. These tiny little seeds are also filled with omega-3 fatty acids, but you don't need to grind them.

Both chia and flax are high in fiber, so be sure to drink plenty of extra water when you eat them. No one tells you this, but if you skip the water you risk worse constipation!

If chia or flax just don't cut it, your local health food store or pharmacy will likely carry the herb senna in tea or pill form. Though senna is a safe over-the-counter supplement that promotes regularity, it is stronger than flax and chia, and should only be used once in a while. You can eat chia and flax daily since they are so good for you.

Exercise is another important and beneficial way to improve digestion . . . and it is free! Exercise promotes peristalsis, which is the movement of food and stool through your GI tract (bowels). Walking just twenty to thirty minutes a day can make a big difference. Exercise not only improves digestion, it can also lift your mood— bonus! Combining exercise with a high fiber, high fluids diet may be all you need to maintain regularity.

If these simple suggestions don't help get things moving, there are of course over-the-counter and prescription remedies available too. Be sure to tell your health care providers all about digestion and discuss any herbs or supplements you plan to add to your regimen.

59.

One-Flavored Zen

DECIDING WHAT TO EAT

Zen offers us the flavor of "the one taste."

THE ONE TASTE is nothing less than the ultimate truth that pervades everything. What is the ultimate truth? Well, that's a bit trickier. As Master Linji (Rinzai) says, the moment you open your mouth you are already way off. Linji preached that words cannot explain, cannot capture, the real nature of the universe. Instead, he taught that you must taste this "one taste" for yourself.

While the "one taste" is something to aim for in terms of Zen practice, it is a real bummer if all of our food has only "one taste." It is common to lose your appetite or have a weird taste in your mouth when you are on chemo. Both of these can make eating more a chore than a pleasure, but it doesn't have to be that way. Sometimes you just have to get a little more creative with your approach to food to get beyond that one (yucky) taste to rekindle your ability enjoy eating.

I once heard cancer chef Rebecca Katz give a talk on

how to make food more pleasurable and palatable during cancer treatments. She recommends making sure that each dish has a number of tastes; all of which make the food more delicious and appealing to our taste buds.

- First, be sure there is some fat in your dish. Stick with healthy fats like olive oil, coconut oil, or ghee (clarified butter). The fat gives your dish better "mouth-feel" and may help rid you of the metallic taste in your mouth, and it could help soothe mouth sores. Plus, healthy fats help you feel fuller longer and help you maintain weight. Try adding a glug of olive oil to your soup, salad, veggies, or a grain-based dish.

- Adding some kind of acid, such as the juice from a lime or lemon, or using some kind of vinegar, will add some flavor complexity to your dish. Acids "brighten up" foods and are often exactly what is missing. Try squeezing the juice from a piece of lime or lemon on your fish, chicken, or tofu, or on a grain-based dish. However, because acids can irritate mouth sores, you may want to skip this tip and instead focus on the other flavor-enhancing techniques.

- Many of us shy away from salt, but our bodies actually need a little bit of salt each day. I recommend sea salt, as it has more natural minerals and no added preservatives or chemicals, unlike commercial table salt. Salt is a flavor enhancer, and even just a small pinch can make a big difference. You can also use soy sauce, tamari, or miso for their salty flavors. I like miso in soups and soy sauce or tamari in my stir-frys. If your food tastes bland, add a pinch of salt to perk up the flavor.

- Finally, almost all of us enjoy a sweet taste. A little bit of sweet can increase your appetite. Stick to more complex-carbohydrate sweeteners, like coconut milk, maple syrup (Grade B is best), fruits, or nut butters. If you are having trouble getting or keeping anything down, apricot juice or coconut water often go down smoothly and easily. Try adding coconut milk to your soup or stir-fry, or make a dressing with peanut butter, lemon juice, soy sauce, and water (to make it the consistency of a sauce) to add to your protein or grains.

Experiment a bit with these ideas to see which foods work for you and which don't. As a general guideline, meals should consist mostly of vegetables, healthy proteins (tofu, tempeh, low-mercury wild fish, chicken, beans, and nuts), whole grains, and a small amount of fruit (berries are best). Minimize red meats, processed foods, dairy products, and refined sugar.

When preoccupied with our health and well-being, we may lose sight of the simple things in life that can lift our spirits a bit, like a delicious well-prepared meal. As if it isn't already hard enough to figure out what we should and shouldn't eat when we have cancer! Try these flavor-enhancing tips to wake up your taste buds so that you can experience more than just one taste at the table.

60.

Flowers Planted When the Ground Is Ready

USING AROMATHERAPY

The Buddha asked Ananda, "When you smell
the fragrance of the sandalwood log, does this fragrance
arise from the sandalwood, from your nose,
or does it arise in the air?"
The Buddha explained to Ananda, "The fragrance,
the nose, and the perception of the fragrance all have
no abode; the act of smelling and the fragrance are
both empty illusions and have no self-nature."

IN THIS PASSAGE from the Surangama Sutra, Buddha was trying to teach Ananda that the distinctions between the sandalwood, Ananda's nose, and the air exist only in the mind. It is impossible to distinguish one of these without implying the other—there is no smelling without a fragrance, no fragrance without air to carry it, and no fragrance if it is not smelled. These, like everything else, are interdependently produced phenomenon. So the Buddha even used the smelling of beautiful smells as a means to help enlighten students of the Way!

It is said that a true master treats each student like a unique flower: each must be approached and tended to in just the right way to grow and bloom. A master cannot force a student to awaken. No one can force a flower to bloom.

As an herbalist, I have used flowers medicinally in my practice for years. When flowers are planted at the right time, when the ground is ready, their colors are brighter and their medicinal properties are more powerful. Essential oils from the most potent flowers contain, in addition to enchanting aromas, therapeutic and potentially medically beneficial plant hormones and chemical compounds.

The quickest, easiest way to get the healing benefits from essential oils is by smelling them. You can either sniff straight from the bottle or buy an inexpensive diffuser to fill a room with essential oil aromatherapy.

Aromatherapy really helps with nausea (I've even seen an oncologist recommend it for that purpose). I've found essential oils to help with anxiety as well. Peppermint, ginger, or cardamom work wonders for nausea. Lavender, melissa (lemon balm), and neroli essential oils all help calm anxiety. I brought neroli to every chemo appointment, and smelling it helped keep me calm for the many hours I was there.

- Try out a selection of essential oils for aromatherapy. Most cities have health-food stores or shops that carry a good supply.
- As you learn which scents work best for you, you will be able to use your creativity to make personalized essential oil blends.
- The little bottle of your personal blend can be carried with you, so you will have it at hand to use as needed.
- Take care to read the ingredients on any essential oils you may purchase, as some companies may dilute the essential oil with cheaper ingredients that have no medicinal value. The best essential oils include only the oil of the particular plant.

Chinese medicine holds that healthily engaging the five senses is the most direct way to affect the spirit. This is likely why we find in most houses of worship music (for the ears), stained glass or beautiful art (for the eyes), incense (for the nose), kneeling pews or meditation cushions (for the body), and food or wine (for the mouth). When you engage your senses, you bypass the thinking mind and go right to the feeling body. Taking into consideration the law of "like treats like," it is as if the "essence" of the plant connects with our own internal "essence."

The use of aromatherapy is a nonverbal, nonintellectual method of affecting your body and mood while calming your spirit. It provides an opportunity to practice presence and mindfulness as you maintain your awareness on the presence and fleeting, interdependent nature of the scent. Plus, focusing on one of your senses helps calm and relax your mind. Try it during your meditation, and see for yourself!

Take time to stop and smell the roses . . . or the ginger . . . or the lavender.

61.

Try Not to Remember What I'm Saying

EATING TO HELP MENTAL FOCUS

A Zen master commanded his students,
"Forget everything I've said."

WORDS ALONE possess little intrinsic value. The master really wants her students to discover their true nature. Students must take action rather than get hung up on their venerable teacher's words.

How we put what we have heard into action is what defines us.

If you have what is commonly referred to as "chemo brain," it may be much easier to forget what someone has said. It can also make us forget what we are supposed to do and when.

Chemo can make us spacey. I remind myself of this when I forget what I am saying as I'm saying it. It can also make us anemic, which makes us even more spacey. Double whammy.

Wait, where was I?

If you have been forgetting where you've put things, or having trouble remembering obvious facts, you too may have "chemo brain." One way to combat this chemo-induced haze is by eating certain foods. A few types of food can help nourish the blood while going through chemo:

- Leafy greens like broccoli, kale, collards, cabbage, Brussels sprouts, and arugula are good, easy-to-find vegetables that are great for replenishing the blood.
- Berries are too, but they should be eaten in moderation because of their high natural sugar content. Berries can always be eaten in combination with nuts in order to offset the effects of the sugar.
- Pastured or organic free-range red meat and liver can be helpful, but these may not be suited to all diets due to high copper or iron content. It is best to check with a good nutritionist if you're thinking of supplementing your diet with meat for nutritional purposes.

However, you can't go wrong by adding a slew of veggies and a handful of berries to your everyday diet. Besides, most vegetables and berries have anticancer properties.

The nutrients in these foods will help boost your blood and could be the thing that helps you to remember where you're supposed to be and when.

If supplementing your diet with these foods doesn't quite give you all the focus you need, try programming reminder alarms on your cell phone, or writing down the important stuff so you don't have to apologize later.

62.

Bitter Taste, Good Medicine

TAKING APPROPRIATE HERBS

"Bitter taste; good medicine."

THE CHINESE LANGUAGE is filled with four character idioms such as this one. The phrase consists of the characters for "bitter," "mouth," "good," and "medicine." Anyone who has ever been to a Chinese medicine herbalist knows how bitter good medicine can be.

If you choose to take herbs during cancer treatment, be sure that you consult with a licensed herbalist. I have seen too many patients spend too much money on herbs that are not right for their constitution, or that are just a bunch of hoopla, despite what advertisements may have claimed.

A licensed Chinese medicine herbalist can customize a formula for you that will minimize the side effects of your treatment while boosting your energy, digestion, and mood. I've used Chinese herbs throughout my entire treatment, and they have certainly made a huge difference. Thanks to the herbal formula I took a few times a day, side effects of my various treatments have been much less than what was expected.

Remember, food is also medicine! If you can't find an herbalist, begin simply with what's on your plate. Bitter herbs, as well as bitter foods, support healthy liver function. Foods with a bitter taste are said to gently cleanse and detoxify the body. Some foods, like dandelion greens, are both a food and an herb. Dandelion greens are very bitter, and they are used in Chinese medicine to gently "clear toxins out of the blood" (detox) and to benefit an overworked liver.

Herbal foods like dandelion greens are completely safe to eat when undergoing cancer treatment. They are high in many types of healthy, beneficial vitamins and phytochemicals. Try adding dandelion greens to your salad or stir-fry. Remember, the greens are very bitter, so taste as you go.

Bitter is better, but a little goes a long way.

63.

A Mosquito on an Iron Bull

PACKING SMALL MEALS

"Like a mosquito on an iron bull" is an old Chinese Zen phrase used to refer to the pursuit of a useless endeavor.

PICTURE A HUNGRY mosquito attempting to dine on the back of an iron bull. Poor little mosquito! He won't be getting any blood. There's no place to take a bite from an iron bull.

Many of us living with cancer may find ourselves feeling like that mosquito: out and about, unable to find any place to take a bite. Most people choose to eat differently and more carefully when dealing with cancer. We might increase our intake of fruits and veggies, or cut back on junk food and soda, for example. If you've been trying to eat healthily, you may have already noticed how difficult it can be to eat well when you are traveling or unable to be home by mealtime. In some cities, finding a restaurant with wholesome food makes you feel like a hungry mosquito on an iron bull.

It is pretty easy to get in the habit of bringing food with you when you know in advance that you will either be hungry or out and about. As I went through chemo, I found that my stomach was happiest when I ate frequently throughout the day. I've yet to find a fellow cancer survivor for whom this wasn't true. If you were not a grazer or a muncher before, you should develop this habit. Coping with nausea or heartburn will require thinking about food more than you did before.

- Start with your weekly shopping list. Load it with as many healthy snacks as you can think of: nuts with raisins or dried berries (no sugar added), whole grain crackers and hummus, and apples with almond or peanut butter. You may be able to find a decent muesli or granola bar that isn't terribly high in sugar. Shoot for less than 5 grams of sugar per bar. If you can find and afford organic foods, choose them to avoid unnecessary chemicals.
- You may find that you stay fuller longer when you combine healthy fats with complex carbs or proteins. A whole grain sandwich of scrambled free-range eggs with avocado and a drizzle of olive oil will keep you full for a good long time. So will whole grain peanut butter toast. Make these ahead of time and take them with you.
- If you don't carry a purse or bag wherever you go, you

may want to get in the habit of carrying a backpack or book bag to facilitate healthy snacking.

Then you can take a bite everywhere you go.

64.

Stick a Needle in It!

FEELING BETTER WITH ACUPUNCTURE

Master Shitou said, "Words alone can't take you to the state of awakened mind. You can't stick a needle in it either."

HIS POINT WAS that no words can convey the experience of awakened mind, which is intangible and without form. There are just some things in life that defy description; phenomena that words can't capture.

Words are likewise inadequate when it comes to describing your body's life-force energy—referred to as *qi* in Chinese medicine—which is also intangible and without form. "Qi" means energy, and Chinese medicine holds that it is the life-force energy within you that supports, sustains, and circulates throughout your body. Qi flows through specific points in the body, which when stimulated with acupuncture will actually "calm the spirit"—the "spirit" being the most intangible part of you; that essential nature to which the mind "awakens."

Unlike the awakened state that Master Shitou refers to,

you can in fact put a needle in qi! When you get an acu-puncture treatment, the needles are used to strengthen, reduce, or move qi energy to promote balance and mind-body health. The results vary from person to person, but most everyone feels better after an acupuncture treatment.

Full disclosure: I am particularly biased here. I've been providing and receiving acupuncture for many years, and I have seen it work wonders time and time again. There are many good studies that demonstrate acupuncture's ability to treat the side effects of cancer treatments. If you are interested in a more in-depth explanation of this heal-ing modality, Stephen Sagar's book *Restored Harmony: An Evidence Based Approach for Integrating Traditional Chinese Medicine into Complementary Cancer Care* is full of easy-to-understand theory and studies of acupuncture.

I myself had acupuncture the day before, during, or a day or two after each chemo treatment. I credit acupunc-ture for helping to reduce nausea, fatigue, and digestive discomfort during chemo. It also calmed my mind and relaxed my body. For me, it was worth it just for its body-mind relaxation effects. Who couldn't use a deep, thera-peutic rest?

- The best way to find a good acupuncturist is to start by asking people you know for recommendations.
- Personalized, individual acupuncture treatments are ideal when you have cancer, as they give you more

one-on-one time with your practitioner, which in turn gives your practitioner a better understanding of the complexities and particularities of your case. However, if money is an issue or you have a good referral, try a "community acupuncture" clinic in your area. Community acupuncture clinics provide less expensive treatments in a group setting.

- If you are thinking, "No way! I'm terrified of needles!" think again. Pretty much everyone comes to acupuncture afraid of needles. Acupuncture needles are as thin as a hair and essentially painless. The acupuncture experience is nothing like the experience of getting a shot at the doctor's office.

This is one of those "Try it! You'll like it!" therapeutic modalities worth leaving your comfort zone for!

Stick a needle in it? Yes, please!

65.

Burning the Buddha for Warmth

KEEPING WARM FOR COMFORT

*During an icy, bone-chillingly cold winter stay
at a temple, Master Tianran burned a wooden
Buddha statue to keep warm.*

THIS ACT was considered sacrilege, and everyone freaked out. They couldn't believe that the master would burn a Buddha statue. Their insight was not as deep as the master's, as they could only see an image of the Buddha, and not the wood.

Since he was absolutely freezing, Master Tianran refused to treat the wooden statue like something other than what it was: wood that could help warm his cold bones. Master Tianran saw through its form and broke with formality. He responded in a spontaneous and Zen-like way to his predicament.

Master Baiyun once said that he had four great vows: "When I'm hungry, I eat; when it is cold, I put on more clothes; when I'm tired, I stretch out and sleep; when it gets warm, I like to find a cool breeze." I really like how he explicitly included the fact that he, too, got cold, and he wasn't embarrassed to put on some extra clothes to keep warm. A great vow indeed.

If you've lost weight, or if you are on certain meds, you may be running cooler than you used to. It may feel odd to always bundle up, but it is important to do so whenever you feel even a little cold. Act like a Zen master and do what needs doing without hesitation! Think of it this way: when we are cold, our bodies use up extra energy to keep warm. Personally, I'd rather preserve my energy for healing!

- One of the best ways to keep the body warm is to keep your neck protected against the cold. A fabulous turtleneck, scarf, or neck gaiter kept in one's bag or car comes in handy for this purpose.
- A warm hat is also a must if you don't live in southern Florida or Mexico.
- Doctors recommend keeping hands and feet warm too to help minimize neuropathy.
- It is harder for a nurse to find a vein if you are cold. See if your doctor has any instant hot packs on hand. You may even want to ask the doctor's office to order them—they're cheap. Place the hot pack over your elbow crease (or anywhere else) before anyone tries poking you. This has worked wonders for fellow cancer patients and myself.
- I have also found that keeping a hot pack over the

infusion site throughout chemo procedures ensures that the fluids aren't uncomfortably chilly as they come in. It just feels better, and the warmth from the hot pack is soothing.

When you are cold, use it as a reminder to channel your inner Zen master. Take care of business spontaneously and without fuss.

As my mother used to say before I left the house, "When in doubt, take a little sweater!"

66.

A Bee Doesn't Return to an Old Hive

STANDING TALL FOR A BETTER VIEW

The past is a nice place to visit, but you can't live there.
Old hives are just that—old.

WHEN A ZEN MASTER reminds you that "a bee does not return to old hive," she is telling you that it is time to move on. She could just say, "Been there, done that," but that would be less poetic.

We should think about how important this mindset is when we feel stuck or feel low. What good does the past do us at this moment? Our goal should be to attend to the present as we work to preserve our future. Being fully present can help reinforce optimism and belief in positive outcomes. What can we do physically to promote greater presence and positive thinking?

Michael Broffman, an amazing Chinese medicine doctor and cancer researcher at the Pine Street Clinic in San Anselmo, California, once gave me some great advice on this subject. He told me to pay attention to my posture and to hold myself as upright as possible. Physically, an upright posture allows us to better see what lies ahead. Energetically, this posture sends an unconscious message that we have places to go and people to see. In other words, we have plans, are heading somewhere, and have a future.

- We can help to develop a greater sense of presence and cultivate positive thinking by paying attention to our posture while we lay down, walk, sit, or stand. These are the four traditional postures that are bases of mindfulness practice in Buddhism.
- Attend carefully to your bodily posture, noting whether you are drooping, slouching, or crumpled.
- Straighten the spine so that the body is well aligned and comfortable.
- Sit or stand as if you are doing so for a purpose.

The more upright you sit or stand, the farther you can see. Try sitting and standing tall and see how different you feel. You'll be amazed. Standing tall helps us to envision where we are headed and to leave behind pining for the past.

67.
Sky Above, Earth Below

TAKING IN THE OUTDOORS

"The sky is above, the earth is below."

THIS ZEN SAYING alludes to what ought to be common knowledge, but sometimes we get so caught up in the daily grind that we don't even notice the wonder of the most common things. When was the last time you got out and actually looked at the sky above or the earth below?

No matter where we live, there are always beautiful views to take in when we go outside. And of course, once we get out and begin to take in our environment, what we see may give us food for thought. Looking around gets us out of our heads, which is usually a most welcome break.

Here's a radical notion: unplug, put on your walkin' shoes, and go experience the nature around you! Even if you live in a big city, you can still find gorgeous nature to experience. Cherry blossom season in New York City, for example, is amazing. Parts of Central Park transform into a flower petal wonderland.

I am spoiled as a San Franciscan, because our weather

tends to be temperate enough to get outside all year round, which also eliminates an excuse to stay inside when I'm feeling lazy. Living in this area, I try to get to the beach and the forest regularly. What types of nature is your area known for?

Even if you do not live in an area that has a mild climate year round, when luck smiles on you and you get a beautiful day, get off your tuchus, get outside, and breathe in the fresh air! For better or worse, your computer will still be there when you get back.

A change of scenery does the mind and body good. When the scenery includes trees, flowers, or a vast and gorgeous sky, even better. As denizens of Earth, we are truly blessed, surrounded by beauty almost no matter where we live. It may have been a while since you've gotten outside to take in and enjoy the scenery.

We all have memories of being truly immersed in the beauty of nature, where birdsong, babbling brooks, and the sound of wind in the treetops greet us. If today is a good weather day, get unplugged and get into nature!

Now is the perfect time to confirm for yourself that the sky is indeed still above and the earth still below.

68.

No Goats or Hounds

ENJOYING CHOCOLATE (YES, CHOCOLATE!)

Master Zhaozhou warned his followers,
"Do not be like goats and hounds."

GOATS AND HOUNDS are always looking for food and putting everything they find into their mouths. If you've been going through chemo, or eating an anticancer diet, chances are that you haven't behaved like a goat or a hound for a while now.

I am a big foodie. And although I don't have much of a sweet tooth, I did find it pretty hard to come up with a satisfying sweet snack that would still be within my pretty strict anticancer diet. You don't have to thank me now, but you'll want to. Why? Because the answer turns out to be fabulous:

CHOCOLATE

Yes, chocolate! Specifically, dark chocolate (no milk). Chocolate contains healthy antioxidants called flavonoids and procyanidins. The EGCG in green tea and resveratrol in red wine are also in the flavonoid family. Milk chocolate and "Dutch cocoa" have less flavonoids. So the darker the chocolate, the better it is for your health.

- Find chocolate that has very few grams of sugar and a high cacao content (70 percent and higher is best).
- The higher the cacao content the more bitter the chocolate will be. Experiment to find the percentage of cacao that suits your taste.
- Chocolate bars usually contain refined sugar, so be sure to read the label to ensure that you don't buy a sugar bomb.
- Eat only a small amount of chocolate at a time—a few squares, not the whole darn bar. This may be tricky at first, but treat the eating of chocolate as an exercise in self-discipline. It gets easier once you get into the habit of eating a small portion of chocolate daily.
- If chocolate is a major weakness for you, it may be best to avoid it altogether.

You may be surprised how tasty and fulfilling just a few bites of good chocolate can be, and you still won't resemble a goat or a hound.

69.
The Taste of Salt

DRINKING HEALTHY SOUP

A monk asked Master Fojian,
  "Why did Bodhidharma come from the west?"
Master Fojian replied, "If you taste vinegar then you
  know sour. If you taste salt then you know saltiness."

THE MONK'S QUESTION is ostensibly about Bodhidharma bringing Zen Buddhism from India to China, but the question implied within it is "What is Zen?" The master refuses to try to put into words that which cannot be put into words: "The Dao that can be spoken of is not the true Dao." The master lets the monk know that he will have his answer only when he experiences his own awakening.

Likewise, I can describe the delicious taste of miso soup, but if you haven't tasted it for yourself, you can't really know what I am describing. Miso has a rich, salty taste. Drinking miso soup is soothing to your stomach. You may have had some at a Japanese restaurant, but it is easier to make at home than you'd think. Once again, you'll never know until you experience it.

Miso soup is a great source of healthy, beneficial nutrients. Miso is a Japanese paste made from fermented soybeans, rice, and sea salt. Soy may not be great for everyone's diet, but it is much more digestible and healthier for you when fermented. If you are avoiding soy as part of your diet, you can also find miso made with other beans.

The best misos are found in the refrigerated section of Asian markets or health food stores. It is best to avoid the room temperature miso stored on the shelves. The misos that are refrigerated are still alive and chock full of healthy probiotics like lactobacillus, which helps digestion. Miso paste also contains isoflavanoids, antioxidants, and minerals, all very helpful and healthy, whether confronting cancer or not.

Miso has been traditionally used in Japan to help the body expel heavy metals. Chinese medicine considers miso to be good for the kidneys because of its salty flavor. Miso is also alkalizing, and studies show that the salt in miso does not raise blood pressure.

And a small amount of miso goes a long way, which makes it an economical health food. There are a wide variety of misos to choose from. Generally, the darker the miso, the stronger its flavor will be. So you may want to begin with a white or red miso before venturing into the darker varieties.

Here is an easy to make, basic miso soup recipe:

- Chop a scallion or two, a carrot, some cabbage.
- Place enough water in a pot to cover veggies and place the pot over a medium flame.
- Place chopped veggies in heating water.
- Add a tiny amount of seaweed (two pieces of wakame or two big pinches of arame).
- Boil the soup until the veggies are cooked and the seaweed softens.
- Distribute the soup into bowls.
- Add about a teaspoon of miso to each bowl, squishing it against the side of the bowl to dissolve it into the soup.

It is best never to boil good miso. When you first make the soup, begin with less miso than you think you will need, adding more to best suit your taste. Build on this basic recipe by adding chopped tofu and/or noodles.

Miso is like Japanese chicken soup. It is good for the soul as well as the belly!

70.
Dragon's Mouth

SOOTHING YOUR MOUTH AND LIPS

Master Tianyi once said, "A handless man
can use his fist. A tongueless man can speak.
If suddenly a handless man strikes a tongueless
man, what does the tongueless man say?"

THIS IS ONE of those typical Zen brain twisters. How can a tongueless man speak? Or a handless man hit with his fist? Sometimes the best answer is no-answer. How do you answer with no-answer? With silence, or maybe even a good shout.

When Master Danxia tested Zhenxie's understanding by asking him to explain what he had heard Master Danxia say in his dharma talk, Zhenxie's response was to be silent. The master replied approvingly, "I'll say you caught a glimpse of it."

In Zen, talk is cheap. Experience and insight are prized over words and descriptions. They say "don't listen to the mouth, watch the actions." I'm sharing this because you may want to keep this in mind if your mouth has become too uncomfortable for random chatter.

Cancer treatment can leave our own mouths feeling scaly, gnarled, and raw. It isn't commonly spoken of, but many cancer patients run into mouth challenges over the course of treatment. Mouth and tongue sores, and chapped and burning lips may leave our mouths seeming like a dragon's mouth.

A chemo buddy of mine and I both had horribly chapped lips since we started treatment. We would compare our thrashed lips to see whose were worse off. Some cancer patients get mouth or tongue sores while others get insanely dry and peeling lips.

Here are a few techniques you may want to try if you have sores in your mouth:

- Gargle with salt water or aloe vera juice a few times a day.
- Brush your teeth with toothpaste that contains salt and baking soda. It may seem strange and funky, particularly if you are accustomed to sweeter toothpaste, but it really does the trick.
- I've found that brushing yields the best results when you rinse your mouth and brush your teeth frequently throughout the day.

- If you can, avoid putting anything on your mouth that contains mint, olive oil, or coconut oil. These can aggravate sore and tender lips.
- Lip balms with a high shea butter or jojoba oil content have proven particularly effective. Calendula and vitamin E have both been proven helpful for lip repair.
- To "seal in" the lip balm so it can help longer, slather basic Vaseline on your lips after you've applied lip balm.
- When venturing outside, apply a high SPF lip balm over the usual healing balm. The combination seems to work better than either alone, and sunburned lips are just the worst!
- Drinking more tea and fluids also helps with dry mouth and lips.

It will likely take some experimenting to see what works best to soothe your dragon mouth. As with Zen koans, there is no "one-size-fits-all" right answer that works for everyone. Often the right answer is to keep your mouth closed, and enjoy the silence.

71.
A Mere Grain of Rice

COOKING SMART

*When Master Guishan noticed that the cook
dropped a rice grain on the floor, he pointed out
that thousands and thousands of other rice grains
could have come from that single grain.*

WHILE IT SOUNDS like he was trying to guilt the cook
(and perhaps a bit of that is in there), the master was
actually pointing out that even something as tiny as a
single grain of rice is valuable and capable of big things.
There are potentially entire fields contained within a single grain of rice. As we care for our bodies while fighting
cancer, it is important to always remember the potential
benefits that even the simplest foods, like rice, can have,
and to take fullest advantage of them.

Veggie stir-fry over brown rice is one of the easiest and
most nutritious dishes we can make. The simplicity of
the dish makes it a great request candidate when friends
or loved ones want to cook for you. In addition to a slew
of colorful veggies, we might include a protein of choice

to make it a well-balanced meal. I like to add some kind of roasted nuts, like walnuts or almonds, for that extra crunch and a little healthy fat to stay full. A splash of ponzu, a Japanese citrus-vinegar-soy sauce, makes everything taste even better.

It may be rarely admitted, but brown rice is hard to digest. Brian LaForgia, my pulse teacher, says that brown rice is hard on the stomach nerves. It contains phytic acid, which can block the absorption of minerals in the rice and have an inhibiting effect on digestive enzymes. White rice doesn't have this issue, but it lacks the beneficial nutrients and fiber that brown rice has. White rice is also not so great for blood sugar.

The best way to deal with the troublesome phytic acid in brown rice is to soak the rice overnight. To make the rice more digestible, lighter, and softer, soak it in water to which a teaspoon or so of apple cider vinegar has been added. The same trick can be used for most grains and beans, which are all more nutritious and digestible after a good soak.

If you go online, you can find many recipes with brown rice as a breakfast porridge, or as a main dish for dinner. Find the ones that look the easiest and most delicious to you.

Any step you take to add nutrients and fiber to your diet can make a huge difference. Just like one tiny grain of rice . . .

72.

Speaking Fire

EASING STOMACH DISCOMFORT

Master Yunmen declared, "A person of the Way
can speak fire without burning his mouth!"

A PERSON OF the Cancer Way, however, doesn't have
it quite so easy. When we speak fire it is likely due to
drug-related heartburn! If we didn't have stomach issues
before treatment began, we likely encounter them once
treatment is under way. Fortunately, there is a really easy
way to prevent heartburn and address a bloated, belchy
stomach.

Licorice herb has been used for centuries to treat heartburn and even mild ulcers. Licorice herb is different from
the red and black licorice vines you may recognize from
the candy aisle, which do not actually contain any real
licorice. While it is certainly possible to find a version of
black licorice that does contain licorice, it still won't have
enough to have the medicinal effects we're looking for.

We can, however, find what we need in a form of licorice called DGL, which stands for "deglycyrrhizinated

licorice." DGL is what you want to ask for at your health food store, preferably as chewable tablets. The glycyrrhizin, which is removed from DGL when it is processed, is a natural chemical constituent of licorice that has been shown to raise blood pressure when taken in excess.

- Chew a couple of not-terribly-tasty-but-effective deglycyrrhizinated licorice antiheartburn tablets about fifteen to twenty minutes before eating. I tried it, and within a day or two the heartburn stopped and didn't come back. Nowadays I take some licorice on occasion as a preventative. The only side effect of DGL is the odd aftertaste that it leaves. But to me that is preferable to speaking fire.

If DGL alone doesn't stop your heartburn, consult a local herbalist or your doctor. I feel that it is important to note that many pharmaceuticals that treat heartburn and ulcers may also cause constipation. Natural aloe juice can also help relieve both heartburn and constipation.

73.
Attaining the Marrow

SOOTHING BROTHS AND STEWS

Bodhidharma, the legendary master who brought Zen
Buddhism to China, asked his students to express their
understanding before he returned to India.

Three of his students expressed their understanding in
turn with words, but the fourth student, Huike, came
forward, bowed deeply, and then returned to his seat.

To the first three students Bodhidharma consecutively said,
"You have attained my skin. You have attained my flesh.
You have attained my bones." When he came to Huike,
Bodhidharma said, "You have attained my marrow."

Bodhidharma then made Huike his dharma heir (successor).

LET'S TALK a bit about marrow, since we're here. Huike
already showed us his mastery of Zen marrow, so let's turn
to more edible matters. The marrow I'm interested in is
the "marrow," or the essence, in our food. You attain the
marrow from your food from slow, long cooking.

If you've been having a hard time eating or digesting
food, a broth made out of long-cooked veggies, or if you

are not a vegetarian, a broth cooked with the bones of whatever meat you use, is one of the best, easiest to digest foods you can put in your belly. Homemade broths are nutrient dense and extraordinarily easy to digest. Stock made from broth contains a wide variety of minerals that are easily absorbed by the body. If you use bones, you also get chondroitin sulphates and glucosamine, both of which are sold as supplements for joint pain (save your money!). The gelatin in the broth can facilitate digestion and the healthy accumulation of digestive juices.

Slow, long cooking breaks food down and makes it much easier to digest. You do lose some vitamins from this cooking method, but you will still get plenty of vitamins from "extracting the marrow" of your ingredients into a nutritious broth or stew.

- As a rule of thumb, try to include a leafy green vegetable or two (bok choy, cabbage, kale, collards, etc.) for vitamins, a few small pieces of seaweed for minerals (wakame or kombu, which you can eat or discard), onions and carrots for vitamins and sweetness, and then anything else you find interesting and delicious.
- Add herbs or spices to taste.
- Choose a protein (tofu, chicken, or fish—beans can be hard on digestion).
- The addition of a grain (such as rice, quinoa, or barley) is optional.

- Throw everything in a pot with cold water and bring to a boil. Leave on simmer for a long time, and do something interesting while it cooks.
- If your soup is vegetarian, cook four to six hours. If your soup has an animal protein with bones, you can cook for twelve to eighteen hours. Twelve to twenty-four hours in a crock pot is a great way to make an easy-to-digest stew instead of a soup.
- Try heartier veggies (like root vegetables) for a stew, otherwise, the veggies will become a dull mush.
- Experiment with amounts of each ingredient; there is no "right amount" of anything in this recipe.

I like to add miso paste to my bowl to make the soup a nutritious superstar. You can also add coconut milk and mild curry powder for a more Indian flavor, or add a dollop of pesto to your stew (at the end) for a more Italian flavor. Some people find it easier to eat the broth after straining out the veggies, or after blending. Again, see what works best for your own belly.

From a Chinese medicine point of view, and in accordance with the law of "like treats like," these broths and stews also help nourish your own bone marrow. We may never attain the marrow of Zen, but the nutrition in food is one kind of marrow we can easily attain!

74.
To Catch a Rabbit

BOUNCING YOUR WAY TO BETTER HEALTH

There is a Zen saying for when you do something
in a less-than-clever manner: Trying to catch a rabbit
by waiting for it to run into a stump.

YOU HAVE TO wonder how many rabbits have been caught using this method. If you think about it, we all kind of do this in our own unique way. We sit around waiting for or thinking about something we want to happen rather than take the action necessary to make it happen. You can think about how great it would be to exercise, for example, but the gym is never going to come to you.

This Zen saying encourages us to go after what we want or need, rather than sit idly by hoping that it will bump right into us. Studies show that cancer patients who exercise do better in treatment and feel better in general. Exercise is a great way to lift your mood, benefit your heart, and promote healthy digestion and elimination. If you have enough energy, it is especially good to exercise the day of chemotherapy treatment and a few days afterward. Apparently this helps the chemo circulate throughout your body. If you've been thinking about exercising, but not doing anything to exercise, or if you haven't had the motivation to exercise, rebounding is an exercise possibility that you may not have bumped into before.

I am a huge fan of rebounding as a primary form of cardiovascular exercise. Rebounding is especially useful when the weather is too nasty to exercise outside. "Rebounding" is the professional term for bouncing on a small, well-built trampoline. With rebounding, instead of trying to catch a rabbit, the jumping and hopping up and down will appeal to your "inner rabbit."

Since there are many cheaply made mini trampolines out there that would prove dangerous to use for regular exercise, I recommend investing in a good quality rebounder that is built to last. You can find a wide variety of rebounders online or at your local health and fitness supply store.

Rebounding is gentle on the body's joints and takes very little skill. Even better, rebounding is amazing for your health. It helps move and cleanse your entire lymphatic system, which is part of your immune system. This helps flush out toxins and cellular waste matter. Rebounding tones and exercises almost every muscle in your body and benefits your cardiopulmonary system (heart and lung function).

Rebounders come with pamphlets and sometimes DVDs that instruct you how to use them properly. Be sure to read or watch these before trying it out. It may take a few tries to get your bouncing balance and coordination. I like to put on some music and bounce to it as if I am almost dancing. I move my arms against gravity to strengthen them while I raise my knees up high with each step for a good stretch and workout.

Of course it is important to get outside and interact with nature, but sometimes the elements are not on our side. The rebounder offers us a great opportunity to put on some fun music and get down with our big bad selves, instead of just sitting around looking out at the rain or snow.

We can bounce and jump ourselves into feeling great even when the weather is terrible! Rebounding gets us off of our good intentions and into an extraordinarily healthful exercise routine.

75.
Sleeping Zen

GETTING ADEQUATE SLEEP

Master Baizhang went into the meditation hall
to find Huangbo fast asleep and another monk
sitting in rigorous meditation. The master
praised Huangbo's Zen and chastised the monk
sitting in meditation.

WHAT WAS Huangbo's trick? Huangbo was able to sleep deeply and fully when he was tired, nothing more, nothing less. He wasn't "trying" to do anything. He was simply being a person asleep. The monk in seated meditation was trying hard to do something and it showed. In Zen, authenticity is valued over adherence to ritual and form.

Sleep is crucial for mental and physical well-being. When we sleep our bodies release healing hormones that help clean up the day's bodily wear and tear. Our mood and energy are also directly affected by how well we sleep. Sleep directly affects our levels of ghrelin and leptin, two ridiculously named hormones that trigger feelings of hunger and fullness. If we don't get enough sleep, it disrupts our appetite big time.

If you've been having trouble sleeping, try taking a bath thirty minutes before bedtime. Put in plenty of Epsom salt and scent the bathwater with a smell that soothes you. If you are in a hurry, simply roll up your pants and soak your legs up to your knees in the bath. When you soak your lower body in hot water, it brings the body's heat and energy down out of your head, which helps you to relax.

To get yourself soundly off to sleep, try the following visualization as you lie in bed:

- Imagine that you are lying in the sand on a beach; the top of your head is oriented toward the ocean.
- Breathe in deeply, all the way down to your belly.
- As you exhale, imagine the warm waves of the ocean washing down through your body—from the head, down through the neck, shoulders, and torso, down through your thighs and calves, and out your feet.
- Relax and inhale deeply, again, imagining a new wave forming and coming toward your head.
- As you exhale, imagine a new, warm, relaxing wave passing through your whole body, washing away any emotional or physical tension as it passes.
- Repeat the cycle until you fall asleep.

The key to success with visualization is consistency. Keep your mind focused on the image of waves of relaxation passing through your body as you allow your breath to grow more natural and deep, and drift away.

You'll be practicing sleeping Zen in no time!

76.
A Picture of Cake

AVOIDING SUGAR

"A picture of a piece of cake cannot satisfy hunger."

THIS ZEN SAYING means that something you look at or study cannot substitute for the experience it describes. Reading and talking about Zen are not the same as practicing Zen. It is much easier to read about something than it is to put it into practice. Practice requires discipline and repetition, and it is through practice that we experience the benefits we have read about.

Eating well is as much of a practice and a discipline as meditation. Luckily, we have many chances each day to make good eating choices. We can collect healthy recipes or anti-cancer diets, but if we don't use them, it is like reading about meditation but never having meditated. We will lack the firsthand experience of what these can acheive.

That being said, even after reading about "anticancer diets," it is often hard to determine which foods to eat and which to avoid, as there are many different schools of thought out there. One food fact agreed upon by the cancer professionals is that when dealing with cancer it is better to learn to look at, rather than eat, a piece of cake. You see, the more sugar you eat, the more insulin you produce. Greater insulin encourages cell growth, including that of cancer cells. Knowing this makes it easier to be disciplined in our eating and to say "no thank you" to a piece of cake.

Sugar is something that most of us consume on a daily basis. When attempting to avoid it, you may find that it is nearly impossible to do so completely. Rather than stress yourself out by attempting to quit cold turkey, you should begin with the more modest goal of minimizing the amount of refined sugar in your diet. If you've already developed a healthy diet, comprised mostly of proteins and complex carbohydrates like beans, vegetables, whole grains, and nuts, it is perfectly fine to have dessert once in a while. Even a small piece of cake, I daresay! The key is to be more aware and thus more disciplined about sugar intake.

- The best desserts, as far as sugar content is concerned, are those made with real fruits, nuts, and whole grains. Fruit pies and crumbles made with whole grain flours are better options than are cakes made with bleached white flour and processed sugar.

- There are a number of natural, nonsugar sweeteners available. Most of us will know honey, maple syrup, and barley malt. On the sweetness spectrum honey is sweeter than maple syrup, and maple syrup is sweeter than barley malt. Despite being natural alternatives to cane sugar, all three of these should still be used sparingly.

- Stevia is an all-natural sugar substitute that doesn't cause an insulin spike, making it perfect as a coffee or tea sweetener. It even comes in convenient little paper packets just like sugar.

- Agave is very popular but should be avoided due to its extremely high fructose content. High fructose content has been linked to insulin resistance, which causes insulin levels to remain unhealthily elevated.

- Take the time to read labels and to note the amount of sugar in the food you consume. You may be surprised to know that granola, commonly thought of as a health food, usually has a ton of sugar. Muesli typically has less. It is ridiculously easy to cut a few grams of sugar from your diet by simply comparing labels.

When it comes to caring for our health, a little bit of sweet will suffice. A major part of making headway, on the Way and against cancer, is to develop the discipline to maintain healthy habits. Healthy eating is just like the practice of Zen: the more you do it, the more you experience the benefits firsthand, which then reinforces your drive to continue to practice. You'll experience and understand that sometimes just looking at a picture of chocolate cake is enough.

V.

Self-Healing Qigong Exercises

77.

Water Wears Down
the Hardest Rock

RELEASING FEAR

A CANCER DIAGNOSIS almost always comes with a heaping scoop of fear. The fear can be ever-present, always lurking just below the surface, it can be triggered by certain events, like a scan, or it can sneak up on us when we least expect it. Either way, fear is an energy vacuum—it can be a real drag.

Yet small steps consistently taken over a period of time, like water wearing a rock smooth, can really make a difference where fear is concerned. One small step we can take is to learn a special technique for releasing fear and tension.

Breathing is the easiest, cheapest, most accessible fear-relieving tool available to us. It is a primal instinct, a natural reflex action that we've been practicing since our first seconds of life in this world. By slowing down the breath, we slow down our minds, relax our muscles, and our fear and anxiety melt away. It is physiologically impossible to have a stress response while breathing slowly and deeply.

Deep qigong (pronounced *chee-gung*) breathing is a quick and easy way to recharge our body's energy levels. It is one of the quickest and most effective ways to saturate our bloodstream with oxygen, delivering its energizing qualities throughout the entire body. The more oxygen we breathe in, the more energy our body can produce for healthy daily living.

The steps to the practice are quite simple and easy.

- Sit down.
- Slowly inhale through your nose. As you inhale, allow your belly to expand and let the air fill your lungs from the bottom to the top.
- Slowly exhale through your mouth, as if blowing through a straw, letting your belly deflate.
- Exhale as slowly and comfortably as you can.
- Inhale a feeling of peace and calm.
- Exhale and imagine blowing fear out through your mouth. Visualize fear leaving your body in the form of a dark mist.
- Continue for as long as time permits.
- Listen to music during the practice if you like.

If you do this for just a few minutes each day, day after day, you can eventually release some pretty wicked fear.

Be like water—strong enough to wear down the hardest rock, little by little, over time.

Inhale, exhale. Inhale, exhale. Drip. Drip. Drip.

78.

Not Found in Understanding

ACUPOINT SELF-MASSAGE FOR CALMING AND SLEEP

THERE ARE MANY questions in life that lack what we might consider adequate answers. For example, "Why me?" is an often asked and rarely well-answered question. Frequently, even the answer to "Why me?" brings another "Why?" and on and on it goes. When living with cancer, it is easy to spend hours stuck in the circle of why.

Sometimes the answers to our questions never come, and we recognize that we need let go of those questions. Sometimes answers do come, many times when we've given up looking for them. Whatever the case, when our minds are too tightly wound and we're trapped in the tightening circle of "Why? Why? Why?" we're apt to lose both sleep and our peace of mind. We need to break the habitual cycles of our monkey minds and just let it go for a while.

One of my favorite practices for resting the analytical mind is an acupuncture point, or acupoint, self-massage technique. It relaxes the body and mind, and is great to do before sleep. Practicing self-massage creates an opportunity to let go of the day's worries and to focus on caring for the body-mind. The practice helps to bring us into the present moment, providing a needed break from our overworked analytical minds.

The acupuncture point that we will massage is located on the bottom of the foot and is called "bubbling spring." It is located where we stand, and so it metaphorically represents where we take a stand in our lives. It reflects where your awareness is right now, right here where you stand.

- Sit comfortably and cross one leg over the other so you can easily reach your foot with your hand.
- Take firm hold of your foot with the parallel hand.
- Use the whole palm (or mostly the heel of the palm if it is easier) of the opposite hand to vigorously rub the entire bottom of your foot, moving your palm back and forth between the toes and the heel.
- Continue rubbing back and forth until both your palm and foot grow nice and warm.
- Once the foot is well warmed, repeat the process with the opposite foot.
- I recommend one hundred vigorous strokes back-and-forth on each foot.
- You can do this anytime you wish, for as long as feels good.

Confronting unanswerable questions is something both students of Zen and cancer patients share in common. Reactions to facing the unknowable can range from fear to frustration to anger to relief to transcendent calm. No matter how skilled we may be at wrestling with the mysteries of "Why?" we all need a break from time to time. Acupoint massage is a proven way to relax the mind and step away from the circle of why.

79.
Monkey Screeches

RELEASING ANGER AND ANXIETY

Do you ever feel like a monkey screeching at the world around you? Or are you the one being screeched at? Or is it just me? Well, Master Zhongyi said that this is how most people interact with their worlds. He described Buddha nature as a monkey inside a room, and outside the room another monkey goes to each of the room's six windows and screeches at the monkey inside. Each time the monkey outside screeches, the monkey inside screeches back.

The six windows represent our six senses. Our senses are how we take in and interpret our world, and then we screech back at the world based on the information we received from our six senses. We may not have the ability to change what comes into our awareness through our senses, but we sure can change how we react to that information. If screeching at the people in your world hasn't gotten you very far—it rarely does—there are far more constructive ways to react to your environment.

You can help change your reality, or at least your interactions, by learning how to therapeutically release pent-up emotional energy, instead of waiting for it to explode in a bout of screeching. Ancient Chinese masters of medicine developed qigong healing sounds as a way to balance emotions and blow off steam.

"Qigong" means "cultivation of energy," and in this case, we will dispel stuck energy to make room for healthy, flowing energy. Healing sounds, also called "healing breaths," help relax and release tension from the body's nerves and tissue. The practice is similar to chanting or the repetition of mantra, only easier.

Before you begin, decide whether you more need to release anger or anxiety. This practice uses the sound HA to release anxiety and the sound SHOO to release anger. You can always do a set of one sound followed by a set of another, if you need to cover both bases.

- Inhale slowly and deeply through the nose, bringing the air all the way down into your belly.
- As you exhale through your mouth, gently vocalize the sound HA or SHOO in a descending tone.
- Let your attention settle on the feeling of the vibration of the sound throughout your body during the long, slow exhale.
- With each inhale, visualize a sense of calm and peace entering your body with your breath.
- With each exhale, feel the vibrations of the sound in

your body and visualize all emotional tension leaving your body through your mouth.

- Repeat the cycle nine times, or in sets of nine, until you feel that the emotional tension has been released.

Healing sounds have been used prescriptively in Chinese medicine since at least 200 BCE—that's quite a few years of clinical trials! See for yourself how freeing it feels to get a break from all of that monkey screeching. Haaaaaaaaaa! Ahhhhhhhhhhh!

80.

When Mind and Body Become One You Are Free

CULTIVATING MEDITATIVE MIND

THERE ARE MANY meditative techniques designed to unify the body and mind. Over the course of many years of study I've come to appreciate the easier ones. When I first began practicing qigong, I tried to find and master the most difficult, complex, and hard-to-learn forms, often with difficult teachers. It took me a while to realize that harder rarely means better.

Now that I've put in years of hard work to master the art of qigong, I have come to respect the power and effectiveness of some of the simplest of its exercises. One of the most potent grounding and centering qigong practices is appropriately called "Buddhist Greeting Posture." You're probably already familiar with the posture of this practice, but you may never have tuned in to its power to bring mind and body together before.

- Sit or stand comfortably.
- If standing, place your feet about shoulders' width apart, keep the spine upright, and the knees unlocked.
- If seated, sit upright in a chair with your feet on the ground, or sit comfortably cross-legged on a cushion.
- Place the palms of your hands together in front of your chest, at the level of your heart, in the gesture of prayer.
- Gently tilt your head down, without bending the body forward. The tilt is minimal; just a slight drop of your chin.
- Let your gaze settle gently on the floor in front of you.
- Drop your awareness into your belly. Allow your relaxed belly to expand with each inhale, to contract with each exhale. Breathing deeply increases the amount of energy-boosting oxygen you take in.
- Keep your awareness focused on the movements of your belly as you gaze downward throughout this practice.
- Quiet your mind and relax your body.
- Continue as long as you like.

The Buddhist Greeting Posture connects the acupuncture meridians in the arms, especially the heart and pericardium meridians. This posture helps relieve nervousness, anxiety, and insomnia. The smooth flow of energy through the heart and pericardium meridians has a calming effect on your mind, as the heart and mind are inextricably linked, both from a Chinese medicine and Western (endocrine) medicine standpoint. Thus, positioning your body in this way enhances the mind-body connection and balances both the mind and the body.

If you are able to maintain your awareness on your belly as it moves with your breath, you become one mind-body circuit, and you experience the peace and calm that naturally arise from this practice.

When mind and body become one, you are free. This freedom is a freedom from feeling like your emotions are in charge of you or rule your behavior. This freedom is your default state, a place of pure awareness where you can witness your emotional "weather" come and go, rather than be swooped up by the breeze of a strong emotion.

When your mind and body are one, your actions are in sync with the peace of mind that is inherent in all of us— the field of pure awareness within which all emotions arise. Unify your body and mind and taste the freedom that has always been yours.

81.

No Consciousness in the Skull

BREATHING TO GROUND AND CENTER

"Empty your head and fill your belly!"

So the Dao De Jing instructs. This cryptic statement has nothing to do with being an airhead with an appetite. It is actually code for an esoteric Daoist alchemical practice.

When we get out of our heads—our skulls—and settle our attention in the belly, body's energy follows the mind to settle there. When we move our awareness away from the frenzied circus of the brain to the settled, even rhythm of deep breathing in the body, everything slows down and the mind becomes clearer. Our "true eye," intuition, opens, and our perspective broadens, shifting from "me, me, me" to "just be, be, be."

The Buddhist notion of awakened mind has nothing to do with the head, either. Master Matsu said that awakened mind is "only peace." So how do we find this peace? Being still and meditating on your breath is the best and easiest place to start. While meditating on your breath does not guarantee awakening, it is said to make you more "accident prone" with regard to waking up. Stilling your body helps still and quiet your mind. Peace will arise within your awareness as you breathe naturally all the way down into your belly.

Belly breathing is the most effective way to calm the mind and to distribute awareness more evenly throughout the body. We can practice it anytime, anywhere.

- Place the palm of your right hand on your chest, and the palm of your left hand on your belly.
- Relax, and breathe naturally through your nose.
- As you inhale, allow the breath to fall all the way down into the depths of your lungs, such that your belly expands, pushing your left hand outward.
- Your chest and right hand should move only after the breath-expanded belly pushes out the left hand.
- As you exhale, empty the lungs from the bottom to the top, such that the expanded belly deflates and the left hand sinks inward.
- Remember to breathe gently, smoothly, evenly, and without force throughout this practice.
- Continue breathing naturally and deeply as long as you like.

Placing the palms of the hands on the belly and chest allows us to more easily focus on the sensation of the belly as it rises and falls. When belly breathing is done correctly, the right hand, placed on the chest, should not rise as much as does the left hand, placed on the belly. Belly breathing can be practiced for a few minutes at a time and as many times a day as feels right.

Buddha belly breathing also provides a quick, effective way to kick in the "rest and digest" relaxation response, which is more easily accessible when we finally manage to get out of our skulls.

82.

Hakuin's Duck Egg

VISUALIZING TO RELAX AND RENEW

THE GREAT ZEN MASTER Hakuin trained with a Daoist qigong master, whom he credited for helping him through a health crisis. Thereafter, Hakuin spent the rest of his life teaching Zen and qigong. The most famous qigong exercise that Hakuin developed involves visualizing magical melting butter the size of a duck egg. Stay with me, it's worth it—Hakuin was no quack! This exercise has a surprisingly calming effect when done with particular concentration.

The practice is best done sitting down with the eyes closed. It is easier to devote all of one's attention to the visualization if a friend reads the visualization aloud. If your phone has a voice memo function, try reading it slowly into the phone's recorder, and listen to the playback of the passage as you practice the visualization.

- Settle into a comfortable, yet stable posture.
- Begin by breathing naturally—slowly and deeply.

- Visualize a warm, round mass about the size of a very large egg, resting on the top of your head. This warm, round "egg" is composed of every healing herb and medicinal substance imaginable. Take a moment to visualize the egg in your mind's eye. Imagine that it begins to emit the smell of fine incense as the heat of your head begins to melt the medicinal, butter-like elixir.

- Feel the warmth of the elixir as it melts down the front, back, and sides of your head, like warm butter melting. Your head grows warm and tingly.

- All the tension and illness in your body dissolves as the medicinal butter melts down your neck, shoulders, and arms, passing to the tip of your fingers and out of your hands. The butter continues to melt down your back, chest, and sides, and then finally down and around your legs, passing to the tips of your toes and out of your feet. Your whole body grows warm and tingly. Take a moment to visualize the feeling.

- Bring your awareness back to the remaining magical healing elixir melting on your head. This elixir melts, passing into your head, through your brain. As the healing elixir descends past your eyes, nose, throat, thyroid, lungs, and heart, feel the warmth as it coats, cleanses, and soothes every organ and every cell. All tension and disease melt away as the elixir melts down and through your body.

- The elixir continues to descend, melting through the digestive organs and reproductive organs, coating, cleansing, and soothing as it fills the urogenital organs, and then melts down into the bones of the legs.
- All remaining tension and illness is washed out, passing through the bottoms of the feet.

Perform this visualization in as much detail and as slowly as possible to reap the maximum benefit. The sequence can be repeated until you feel completely calm and energized.

83.
Take What I Say as Dirty!

PURIFYING YOUR ENERGY

Master Zhaozhou admonished his disciples
not to assume that his words were clean, but to
"Take what I say to be dirty."

HIS DISCIPLES interpreted this statement in various ways, depending on their degree of insight. In order to receive the teaching cleanly or freshly, his disciples needed first to dispel the staleness of clinging to Zhaozhou's words. He was simply challenging them to seek and do for themselves rather than rely on hearsay about his own insight. That is the sign of a great teacher indeed.

In qigong we say "Don't put clean water in a dirty glass." This expression similarly refers to the value of cleaning out old, stagnant energy in the body before filling it with new, fresh energy for healing and calm.

"Cleansing Qi" is a powerful qigong exercise that cleanses the body of stagnant energy and washes the body with the fresh energy all around you. It is a perfect exercise for when you feel sluggish, beat, or emotionally overwhelmed. Cleansing the qi helps to move heavy energy through you and to harmonize you with your environment.

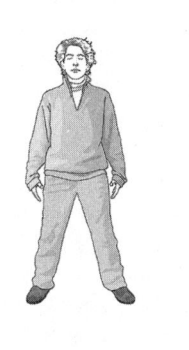

- Stand with your feet shoulder-width apart, with your arms relaxed at your sides. Unlock the knees. Breathe slowly and deeply down to your belly.

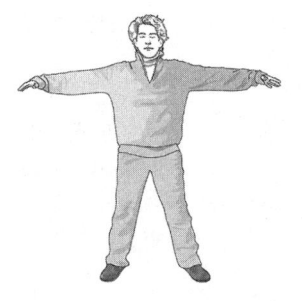

- As you begin a long inhale, raise your arms out to your sides with the palms facing the earth, until they reach shoulder height.

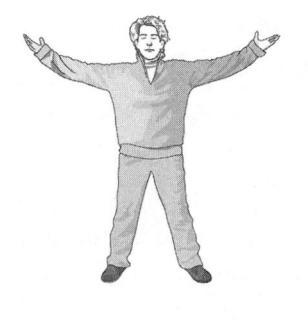

- As you continue to inhale, turn your palms upward toward the sky and continue to raise your arms over your head.

- When your arms are almost straight up, with the palms facing each other, exhale slowly and lower your hands down in front of your body, the palms facing the ground and the fingertips pointing toward each other.

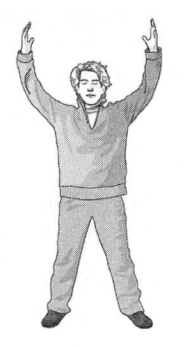 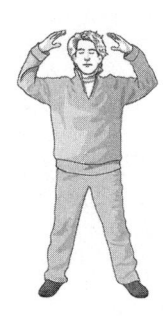 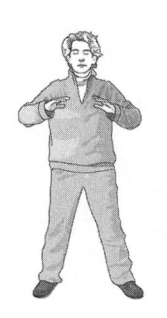

- Return your arms to the relaxed position at your sides where you began.

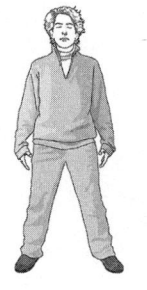

- Repeat at least six to nine times, at any time of day.

Visualization may be added to enhance the exercise. On each inhale, imagine that your palms gather fresh, clean energy from all around you—from deep within the earth and from high above in the sky. On each exhale, imagine that the clean energy rinses the entire inside of your body, washing old energy or stuck emotions out, down through the bottoms of your feet into the ground.

Think of Cleansing Qi as your own portable energy (qi) shower.

84.

Heaven and Hell

CREATING AN ENERGETIC BOUNDARY

A monk asked Master Yangshan,
  "What is the difference between heaven and hell?"
The master simply drew a line in the ground.

THE MASTER gave the monk a clear lesson that we all determine for ourselves what is heaven and what is hell—a difference as arbitrary as where we draw the line in the sand. Heaven and hell are, in the end, what we make them out to be.

We have all experienced how quickly a situation can turn from heaven to hell when we lose our cool. We may be having a seemingly heavenly experience, and then that particular person or annoying thing suddenly appears, on purpose or by chance, and we're not having fun anymore.

In qigong we have a technique to prepare ourselves for inevitable hardship or for situations we expect to be difficult. We use a visualization technique called an "energy bubble," which I've used and taught in many variations for over a decade. This practice is best done before one enters a challenging encounter. It can be done before you leave the house, while you are on the subway, or in your car, for example.

- You can do this sitting in a chair, on a cushion, or standing with your feet shoulders-width apart, knees unlocked.
- Close your eyes.
- Slow and deepen your breathing until you feel your body relax.
- Visualize a bubble around your entire body. Take as much time as you need to mentally create a thick, protective bubble that completely surrounds you.
- In your mind's eye visualize all the qualities you wish to infuse into the bubble.
- Give the bubble a color and texture to solidify the visualization. I like to visualize the bubble like soft, thick, clear glass around me, as if it is freshly blown glass that stays soft and malleable. You can also see it as a golden ball of rippling energy, or as white light surrounding your whole body. Experiment to find what visualization works best for you.
- Now tap in to your sense of personal power and strength: remember a time when you did something that made you feel strong and powerful, and use the feelings of strength and power that arise from that memory. Feel that power and strength fill your body, and then visualize it expanding through your body

to fill the entire inside of the bubble. We all have special gifts that make us unique and wonderful. Use what is special about you and let it fill your bubble.

- Before concluding, take an extra minute to solidify this energy bubble visualization infused with your personal power. Do this by seeing the entire bubble in your mind's eye—it's shape, color, texture—completely surrounding your whole body. Again tap in to your inner strength and recall all of your most amazing qualities and allow the feelings that arise to fill the bubble.

- Carry the sense of being surrounded by the bubble with you as you conclude the session.

Visualizing the energy bubble is a great way to keep yourself grounded, rooted, and firmly centered in situations that are out of your control. Keeping yourself mentally grounded and balanced allows you greater control over where the line is drawn in the sand. It may even help you not to draw a line at all.

85.

Draw Your Bow
Before the Thief Runs

STRETCHING FOR BRAVERY AND ENERGY

In Zen, timing is everything. You must be fully present and aware to respond appropriately to whatever is in front of you. If you miss the right moment to take action, historically you would likely get whacked with the "encouragement stick." Zen requires bravery, especially when engaging in koan training with your teacher. You are expected to respond to a koan question immediately, spontaneously, and authentically with no hesitation. If you hesitate even for just a second before responding, you are said to have drawn your bow after the thief has already started running away. Too late!

If you wanted to stop a thief, would you draw your bow while the thief was nearby and within range, or would you wait until the thief ran away? A brave archer draws her bow at just the right time, or at least as close to the right time as she can.

Are people telling you to be brave? That can be either

encouraging or feel like a command, depending on your mood and the situation. There is a time to be fierce and a time to just crumple into a ball and cry. Now is the time to practice being a brave warrior (unless you are reading this while in a crumpled state and can't muster up the energy, in which case, come back soon!).

This qigong exercise turns you into an archer and puts you in a power stance to help you tap into your inner strength. Drawing the Bow has been practiced at the Shaolin Buddhist temple for centuries in China, and the Shaolin monks are known for their incredible martial arts skills and strength. I can't describe the powerful feeling you get when you take the archer's stance. As with Zen, you just have to experience it yourself to know.

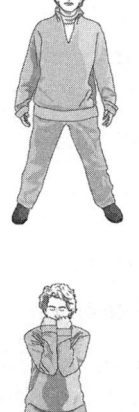

- Stand with your feet shoulder-width apart and unlock your knees.

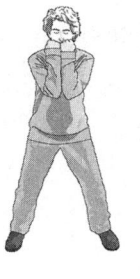

- Put your elbows and wrists together in front of your chest so that the insides of your wrists and forearms and elbows are all touching if possible. Make fists with your fingers facing your face (so you can see your nails).

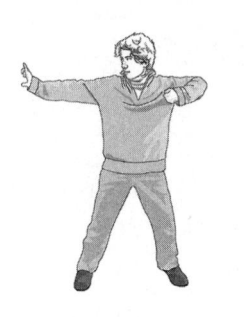

- On an inhale, look over your right shoulder as your left hand pulls an imaginary bow toward the left and your right arm extends out to your right at shoulder's height.

- The right hand's thumb and index finger form a backward L. Tuck the rest of your right fingers into a fist. Try to point your index finger toward the sky with your right arm fully extended out to your right side as you look over your right hand.
- During that same inhale, your left hand is in a fist, pulling a bow with your left shoulder relaxed and your left forearm parallel to the ground.

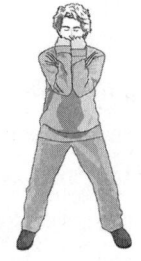

- On the exhale, bring your elbows and forearms back together to starting position and turn your head forward.

- Inhale and now pull the bow with your right arm as you turn your head left and look over your left arm and hand, which are extended to your left with the thumb and index finger making an L.

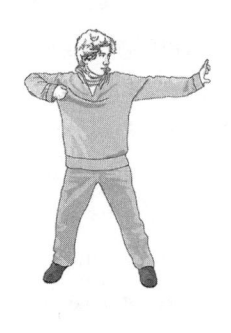 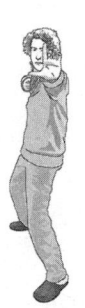

- Exhale your hands back to starting position as you face forward.

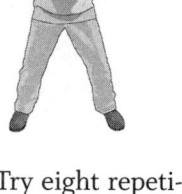

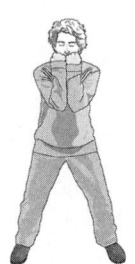

- Repeat as desired. Try eight repetitions to each side to start, and work your way up from there.
- End by returning to the relaxed opening position from which you began, with your arms at your side.

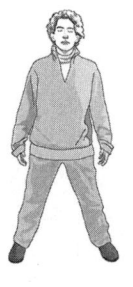

Once you get the movements down you can start to focus on cultivating a feeling of bravery and strength as you inhale and draw your bow. The truth is that these movements naturally bring out the feeling of being a master archer. It takes three to five minutes of practice for me to experience a sense of strength, power, and groundedness from this exercise.

If you are up for a bit more of a challenge, I like to take a wider stance and slightly squat as I do this exercise. The upper body remains upright and there are no changes to what you do with your arms. The only difference is that your legs are in a squat, so they get a stronger workout. I also like the feeling of being lower to the ground in such a stable and strong position.

Drawing the Bow is also a fabulous, quick, pick-me-up, as it helps improve the flow of energy, blood, and body fluids through your entire upper torso. It also opens your chest and benefits the lungs, heart, wrists, and neck.

I can hear Master Baijiao's words now: "If you are brave, come out of the womb roaring like a lion!"

86.

Dragging a Cat

COPING WITH PAIN

I have often heard the maxim "Pain is inevitable, but suffering is optional" around Zen centers. I can see how that might seem cold or stoic, and it is of course easier said than done. But learning how to "be with" when we have no other option is a Zen skill that can really come in handy when it comes to pain. Suffering occurs when we resist what is true and real and here, and what is more true and real and here than pain?

During a particularly long, painful meditation session, we may tell ourselves to "be the pain." This sounds a bit simplistic, but what we mean is to tell ourselves to stop fighting; stop resisting the reality that we have pain, and see how well we can function along with it for the time being. Fighting pain is like dragging a resisting cat across a carpet. The cat is miserable and the carpet gets shredded.

My teacher's teacher used to say that Zen without pain is like noodles without soy sauce. Pain gave his Zen a bit of flavor. When you're a tired cancer patient, pain doesn't seem to add any flavor. It just makes you more tired. So what can you do?

For starters, I would like to say that I am not an advocate for foregoing medication to manage pain. Nevertheless, there are times when pain can be more or less manageable without medication and a simple technique like the following can be useful. Even when pain is sufficient enough to warrant medication, this technique will be helpful during the period between taking the pills and when they kick in.

To "become the pain" we must first surrender. We surrender by relaxing. We relax by further releasing tension from our bodies with each exhalation. This is the key step. As the body relaxes, the entire nervous system relaxes.

Do a quick mental scan of all the major joints, organs, and masses of tissue in your body, from your head down to your fingers and toes, paying attention to each piece to see if you can relax and release it even more. Perform the scan by slowly moving your attention throughout your entire body.

Once you have become as physically relaxed as you can in the face of the pain, begin the following potent qigong breathing technique:

- Close your eyes and continue to relax your body as much as possible.
- Inhale through your nose. As you inhale, allow your belly to expand and let your lungs fill from their

bottoms to their tops. Breathe deeply, slowly, and without force.

- Purse your lips as if blowing through a straw, and exhale fully by blowing through your mouth as if blowing through a straw.
- Concentrate on the feeling of each muscle relaxing and releasing, from your head down to your feet, letting the body relax further with each exhale.
- Continue breathing in through the nose and out through the pursed lips as you move your attention slowly down through your entire body, including your arms, legs, hands, and feet.
- Focus on releasing a little bit of the resistance to and resentment of the pain with each out breath.
- Continue to breathe slowly and deeply, in through the nose, out through the mouth, while releasing a little more pain, tension, and resistance with each exhale.

Tackling pain comes easier for some than others. If this technique reduces pain or helps your pain become more manageable, great! If it doesn't, please don't torment yourself. Pain is pain, and fighting it will needlessly tire you. No need to drag a cat across the carpet!

In Memoriam

A Wave Rises Out of the Ocean

**IN MEMORIAM DAJU HUIHAI SUZANNE BETH FRIEDMAN
(JUNE 21, 1968–MARCH 3, 2014)**

I ENCOURAGE YOU ALL to take a breath—for Suzanne, for you, (for me,) for the earth, the sky, the sun, and the moon.

I would like to write here of Suzanne's life mostly by talking about her death. Over last few days, I sat with her thinking, "She taught me how to live, and now she is going to teach me how to die," and boy, did she ever! Suzanne's death was the most beautiful experience I could have possibly imagined. And it was time for her to go.

Suzanne told me that after death, she did not want us to just "celebrate her life" but to contemplate her death. A poem on her wall at home says:

> Die while completely alive,
> Be completely dead.
> Then do as you will
> and all is fine.
> (Shudo Bunan Zenji)

Suzanne was a fighter, a healer, a guide, a lover, and a teacher. She never complained, and though she lived with so much discomfort for so very long, she always said, "At least I am here to bitch about it!"

Joy and laughter were constant in our home and with her family and friends, and we can all speak to her sense of humor. She thought of others before herself. She loved teaching and loved her students. When a dear friend asked her just a couple of weeks ago what she learned while teaching the last three weekends in a row, her response was "I learned that I can still teach no matter how bad I may be feeling."

"Many great teachers are leaving the earth at this time" was a message that came through to Anna Dorian from her spirit guides and in regards to Suzanne, and this is so, so true. Teaching for Suzanne was her art, her service, her love. She taught Dharma and was deeply committed to that path. She taught medical qigong, Chinese medicine theory, and more. But what she really taught all these years was how to love and see your own essence—and to work from there.

No matter who you think you are or how messed up you think you are or where your life has taken you, you have your gift to offer, and you cannot deny the world that gift. She believed in you, she saw you, and in her funny, direct, and loving way, she begged you to see yourself too.

I've been through a lot with Suzanne in our short years together. I have seen her will to live be stronger than any other person on this earth. She took her own path and walked her own walk.

A week ago from today, on Friday night, I sat with her and the hospice doctor. She was in respiratory distress, uncomfortable and unable to hold her head up or to breathe easily. For the first time ever, I heard her say, "I just can't function like this for much longer," and she expressed the wish just to be comfortable. And that was the first time I had heard her say she was ready to die.

On Saturday, in a miraculous transfer, her sister and I got her up, to the bathroom, and guided her into the yellow room in our house where the shrine of all the countless buddhas, cards, offerings, and light awaited her. In that moment of transition, she had what we call in Chinese medicine the last surge of yang, or false yang, where she became animated, alive, and alert. She sat up in bed, smiled, and spoke to all of us, gave her dad a hug, and told her mom on the phone, "I love you, Mama."

She registered the room, the people, the sky, the buddhas, and her favorite image of "Thanatopsis, Contemplations on Death," who no doubt helped guide her through the dying process. And then moments later, she returned to her inner world.

On Sunday, she was mostly subtle, contained within her own mind, with gentle soft mumblings, occasional utterances that we could understand and many that we could not. Early that morning I read her words from Junpo, her beloved Dharma teacher, that read, "Let go now beloved, sunyata is ever waiting. Enough pain, enough suffering."

And I read her this poem from Enkyo Roshi:

> The wave rises out of the ocean,
> takes its own shape, its own speed,
> its own color, and then, after its crest, slowly,
> kindly, finally, returns to the vast ocean.
> Suzanne, such wild clarity, such brilliance!
> What a life! What passion for Dharma!
> What love you found!
> Such a bond, not always easy, yet tender,
> Oh!
> One by one, the waves come in,
>   and then return, return.

She sat with this a while, quiet, and then in a clear, soft, quiet voice said to me, "I will return to the vast ocean."

Later that day, several people stopped by to offer prayers, the Heart Sutra, blessings, love, touches, kisses, and goodbyes. She had the sound of the ocean playing in the background her last twelve hours throughout the night, guiding her to the return to the great vast ocean that she is.

On Monday morning, March 3, I sat with Suzanne from 3 to 5 AM holding her hand and foot, giving her liquid medication every hour in her cheek with help from my brother, Tom. Lung time, from 3 to 5 AM, was always the hardest time for Suzanne, but this morning was different. She was at peace, silently breathing, soft and shallow breaths.

I asked her permission for the honor of taking her pulse during this time. At 4 am, it was floating and pounding, with no root, but with some force (likely from the medication). Her pulse was fast at about 118 beats per minute.

At 4:55 AM, everything changed. Her pulse was now sixty beats per minute and very soft and weak. I turned to Robert, Suzanne's dad, who was sitting there quietly with me, and said, "It's time to gather people; her death is near."

So our loving team came in the room, silent and peaceful, holding her hand, stroking her back and head, kissing her kepi, expressing our love, and letting her know it was okay to go.

We whispered, "Let go, let go, let go," "Go into the light," "It's okay," "The great ocean awaits you."

Forty minutes later, with her head peacefully lying on a pillow and the most serene expression on her face, her breath slowly drifted off like a gentle breeze. She died with a flower in her palm, hand resting on a Hollow Bones Sutra book, with love surrounding and allowing her to go.

I had known throughout the night that she would die with the rising sun. Moments after her last peaceful breath, at 5:40 AM, the sun rose, and the most brilliant purples and pinks filled the sky. It was the most magnificent sight. We opened the sliding glass door and let the birdsong in. She heard them sing. I know she did. And she loved it.

Suzanne died on the third day of the third month, and it took her three days to die once it was clear this was her time. She had her official diagnosis of cancer for four years and six days, and while there was so much challenge and difficulty, there was always so much joy. I am forever thankful to her for the joy and love we shared and the joy and love I witnessed in her sharing with everyone.

I feel a great honor for having been able to help facilitate and witness Suzanne's profound and peaceful death. It feels like the greatest accomplishment of my life, and I could not have done it without the tremendous support, teamwork, and love of Suzanne's family, my family, and my dear, dear friends. You know you who are, and thank you. Thank you for helping to give Suzanne this most precious and final gift. She, I know, is eternally grateful.

With that, I will end with a haiku poem I gave to Suzanne years ago.

No flower can stay
Yet humans grieve at dying
The red peony
(Edith Shiffert)

Thank you, Daju Suzanne Friedman, you now are alive for me in every flower I see.

I love you.

Words delivered at the funeral
services of Daju Suzanne Friedman
By Suzannah M. Stason
March 07, 2014

Suzannah M. Stason is a licensed acupuncturist, herbalist, and medical qigong therapist in San Francisco, CA.

About the Author

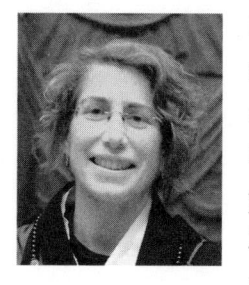

HAVING FIRST ENCOUNTERED Zen at the Nagaoka Zen Juku, a Rinzai Zen monastery in Japan, Daju Suzanne Friedman went on to become a Zen priest in the Hollow Bones Rinzai Zen Order in the U.S. She was an acupuncturist, herbalist, and a doctor of medical qigong therapy. Daju was a professor of qigong and Daoist spirituality at two Chinese medicine schools and led Hollow Bones Zen meditation retreats and services throughout the San Francisco Bay Area. She was an award-winning haiku poet and an author of several medical qigong books. She also played the *shakuhachi* (Japanese Zen bamboo flute) as a meditative practice. Daju once survived cancer and was an incredible inspiration to many. She passed away peacefully at home in March of 2014.

About Wisdom

WISDOM PUBLICATIONS is the leading publisher of classic and contemporary Buddhist books and practical works on mindfulness. Publishing books from all major Buddhist traditions, Wisdom is a nonprofit charitable organization dedicated to cultivating Buddhist voices the world over, advancing critical scholarship, and preserving and sharing Buddhist literary culture.

To learn more about us or to explore our other books, please visit our website at www.wisdompubs.org. You can subscribe to our eNewsletter, request a print catalog, and find out how you can help support Wisdom's mission either online or by writing to:

Wisdom Publications
199 Elm Street
Somerville, Massachusetts 02144 USA

You can also contact us at 617-776-7416 or info@wisdompubs.org.

Wisdom is a 501(c)(3) organization, and donations in support of our mission are tax deductible.

Wisdom Publications is affiliated with the Foundation for the Preservation of the Mahayana Tradition (FPMT).

Hidden Spring

A Buddhist Woman Confronts Cancer

Sandy Boucher

224 pages, $16.95

"An unflinching, poignant, inspiring account."—*Booklist*

How to Be Sick

A Buddhist-Inspired Guide for the
Chronically Ill and Their Caregivers

Toni Bernhard

Foreword by Sylvia Boorstein

216 pages, $15.95

"Full of hopefulness and promise… this book is a perfect blend of inspiration and encouragement."
—*The Huffington Post*

Mindfulness Yoga

The Awakened Union of Breath, Body, and Mind

Frank Jude Boccio

Foreword by Georg Feuerstein

368 pages, $19.95

Editor's Choice
—*Yoga Journal*

Sit with Less Pain
Gentle Yoga for Meditators and Everyone Else
Jean Erlbaum
Foreword by Frank Jude Boccio
200 pages, $19.95

"A very useful book, which could benefit many."
—*Wildmind Buddhist Meditation*

Veggiyana
The Dharma of Cooking:
With 108 Deliciously Easy Vegetarian Recipes
Sandra Garson
320 pages, $19.95

"Pure and simple ingredients, brilliantly easy recipes,
and a liberal serving of Dharma will nourish
the body of wisdom well past mealtime."
—Karen Maezen Miller, author of *Hand Wash Cold*

.